BURNED OVER!

BURNED OVER!

The Survival of Montana Firefighter
Dan Steffensen

Written by

A.J. Otjen

2023 Library of Congress Award-Winning Author

sweetgrassbooks
an imprint of Farcountry Press

Library of Congress Control Number: 249037

ISBN 978-1-59152-345-1

© 2024 by A.J. Otjen

Design by Sue Murray

For more information or to order extra copies of this book call Farcountry Press toll free at (800) 821-3874 or visit www.farcountrypress.com

Front Cover: Britannia Mountain Fire eight miles NW of Wheatland, Wyoming. Pictured are Dan Steffensen, Hank Rae, and Wyoming Hotshots. Courtesy of Kyle Miller Photography.

Back Cover: Courtesy of Kyle Miller Photography.

s⚘eetgrassbooks
an imprint of Farcountry Press

Produced by Sweetgrass Books

PO Box 5630, Helena, MT 59604; (800) 821-3874; www.sweetgrassbooks.com.

The views expressed by the author/publisher in this book do not necessarily represent the views of, nor should they be attributed to, Sweetgrass Books. Sweetgrass books is not responsible for the author/publisher's work.

Produced and printed in the United States of America

28 27 26 25 24   1 2 3 4 5

Dedicated to
Red Lodge Fire Rescue,
the Salt Lake Unified Fire Authority,
and the University of Utah Health Burn Center.

In loving memory of
Kelly Steffensen

Contents

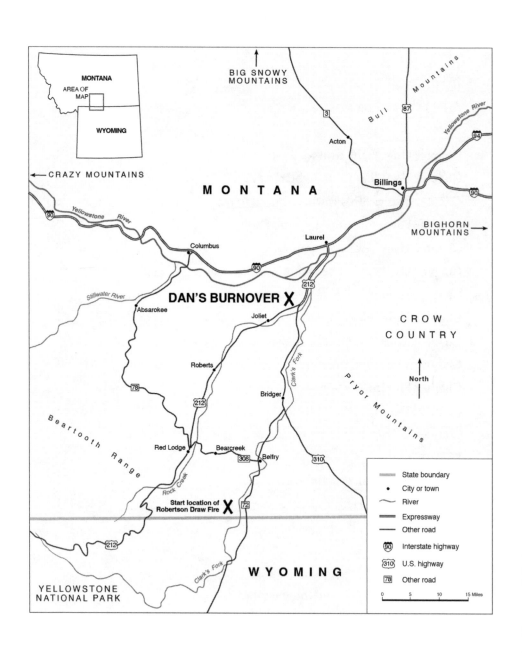

Author's Note

Dan and I chose the title *Burned Over!* because those are the two most terrifying words for a wildland firefighter to hear. Everyone heard it on the radio that fateful day—along with "need help," which is precisely what Red Lodge and Utah gave Dan and his family.

When I first met Tom Kuntz, chief of Red Lodge Fire Rescue in Red Lodge, Montana, he asked if I thought a fire author should write this "amazing story."

I thought he might be right. Dan asked me to help him tell this story. He read a children's book I wrote and published with the artist Kevin Red Star, who also lives near Red Lodge. It was Dan's confidence in me that kept me going.

This is not just a fire story. It's a human story about the town of Red Lodge, Montana, in what is still called the "Summer of Hell," when Dan's burnover was just one of many horrific tragedies. It is about firefighters and their families and how they responded when, as Dan says, "Shit happens fast."

I wrote this as a narrative non-fiction, often intruded upon with a journalistic style, including direct quotes from the people there. Most were too emotional to find the words to describe their feelings about the events. But everyone generously shared their time and memories, helping me to portray the story as it unfolded.

I use titles such as Chief or Captain mainly when the scene shows them on duty. But I mostly use first names, as this is a family, and when I interviewed them, that is how they referred to each other.

Though there may be challenging pieces in the following pages, to quote Tom: "We sleep well at night because 1) Dan knew what he was doing and did the right thing in a bad situation that was not preventable; 2) our organization did an incredible job to support him and his family; 3) we are fortunate that Dan is such a tough guy."

By telling this story, Dan is saying "thank you" for the Herculean effort of the thousands of people who worked to save him. His story is merely the thread that reveals how often these good people step up to greatness.

Acknowledgments

Thank you to my friends who reviewed early drafts to help point out my foibles: Cindy, Sarah, Jana, Anne, Renee, and Deborah. Also, Captain Will Bernard graciously reviewed my firefighting accuracy. My dear longtime friend Patricia Ridge Bradley designed the cover. Dan's friend Kyle Miller, photographer and Wyoming Hotshot, is responsible for the cover photography.

Thank you to editor LA Eaton, as well as the entire team at Sweetgrass Books.

Thank you, Dan, for asking me to be the one to tell your story.

Especially, thank you to the people below, who contributed their time and memories to help Dan share his remarkable journey.

Family
Dan Steffensen
Kelly Steffensen
Cindy Northey
Hannah Langenbahn
Will Steffensen
Susie Steffensen
Mandy Peck
Margot Dickinson

Red Lodge Fire Rescue members
Chief Tom Kuntz
Deputy Chief Tim Ryan
Assistant Chief John Trapp
Assistant Chief Jim Avent
Captain Tyler Rae

ACKNOWLEDGMENTS

Captain Will Bernard
Lieutenant Amy Hyfield, Public Information Office, Firefighter, EMT,
    SAR
Firefighter Katy Hedtke
Firefighter Danny Johnson
Firefighter Scott Wilson
Sarah Ewald, Foundation Director, Firefighter, EMT
Ruth Bilyeu, Community Care Director, Senior EMT
Cathie Osmun, Retired Red Lodge Fire Rescue EMT

Salt Lake Unified Fire Authority
Wildland Division Chief Anthony Widdison
Assistant Chief Riley Pilgrim
Chief Dan Petersen (Ret)
Battalion Chief Dusty Dern
Behavioral Specialist Captain Layne Hilton
Honor Guard and Firefighter Captain Jared Wayman

University of Utah Health Burn Center
Nurse Erik Mandeen
Program Coordinator Kristen Quinn
Doctor Callie Thompson
Charge Nurse Emily Pascua

Montana DNRC/Southern Land Officer Jeff Brown
Chief Melvin Hoferer, Joliet (MT) Volunteer Fire Department
Chief Mike Maltaverne, Teton County Fire & Rescue (ID)
Marla Frank, Joliet (MT) Paramedic
Doctor Kathi Theade, St. Vincent's ER
Larry Vukonich
Kari Boucher-McCleary

All other sources are noted.

Since 1910, the year the Great Fires of Idaho and Montana killed seventy-two, over nine hundred wildland firefighters have died fighting fire. Most of them burned to death. And burning on a mountainside is a hellish death. When firefighters die in a forest fire, they burn from the inside out. The fire sets up its prey before it arrives by emitting a radiant heat that cooks the air. Trapped firefighters hysterically inhale the on-fire oxygen, which melts their lungs before the ravaging crematorium consumes their bodies. Imagine moving closer and closer to a whistling kettle, through its steam, until finally, your lips wrap themselves around the spout, and you suck in with deep and frequent breaths.

Matthew Desmond, *On the Fireline*

CHAPTER ONE

Tight-Knit

It would come to be known as the Summer of Hell.

At the base of a trailhead, a tourist preparing for a hike or a family from out of town enjoying a picnic by Rock Creek wouldn't be aware of the havoc that Mother Nature caused in Red Lodge, Montana, in 2021.

Aspen and spruce trees dot between the lodgepole pines rooted on towering mountains framed against blue skies. The valley inspires spirituality for those who pray. The smell of pine, juniper, and sage, especially after it rains, is nature's intoxicating perfume. It creates a permeating incense, inviting even agnostics to believe in a higher power.

Trailheads open the door to the wilderness in the Beartooth Mountains, whose heights deliver vistas of other mountain ranges miles away. A paintbrush of color reveals vast prairies separating the snow-capped ranges. The Crazy Mountains, the Big Snowies, the Absarokas, and the ancient Pryors, where the wild horses run free, are all worth the climb.

As visitors breathe in the fresh, crisp air, they are unburdened by images of charred faces and burnt flesh. They don't hear a two-way radio crackle before a voice comes over it, alarmed by a burnover. They don't have to experience the anguishing sounds of a firefighter whose skin is melting in an inferno. These visitors most likely know little about this land, where fires maim, kill, destroy vegetation, and break families apart. But the residents of Red Lodge do.

Situated on the northern edge of Yellowstone National Park, Red Lodge is about sixty miles south of Billings, in the heart of Apsaalooke Crow country.[1] It is a ski town in the winter, with a mountain terrain mostly left ungroomed, making it a hidden jewel for skilled skiers. In the summer, millions of tourists drive down the main street of Broadway towards the Park, stopping for a Montana cowboy hat or moose sculpture to take back home.

For the locals, at home on the well-known wilderness trails for their cross-country treks on foot, skis, or horses, the town is an entire community where everyone knows your name. It's a tight-knit group of people who depend on each other for survival. Their home is heaven, surrounded by forest and grass fuel, just waiting for someone to strike a match. The price of living in paradise is the understanding that things can change to hell in a heartbeat.

The infinite Montana sky could be as clear and blue as a painting, and then a thunderhead cloud might grow so tall in the distance that it looks like a cottonwood tree has sprung from the ground, bleached white against the cyan sky. Its majesty stuns the eyes and hides the dangerous outflow boundaries that can quickly alter wind direction by 90 to 180 degrees. The roar of that wind is the last thing a firefighter may hear before he dies.

Montana is a firefighter's wide-open experiential classroom. Weather can change fire behavior in seconds. Most Montanans know how to identify rapidly changing weather by examining swaying trees or observing smoldering fires. Firefighters are trained to study lenticular clouds, fast-moving clouds, cold fronts, cumulonimbus clouds, dust clouds, and sudden, shifting winds. These are signs of atmospheric instability, portending things like thunderstorms and downdrafts exceeding sixty miles per hour, which can blow in from anywhere, especially during hot, dry days.

This is the same terrain that trapped thirteen Forest Service smoke-jumpers in Mann Gulch near Helena, Montana, in 1949 and fourteen in the South Canyon Fire near Grand Junction, Colorado, in 1994. Fire can crawl like a snake through varied and rough terrain, hiding as it grows. Deadly sculptures such as steep chutes, chimneys, passes, saddles, narrow and box canyons surround Red Lodge.

Nature can alter fire behavior faster than a firefighter has time to think. Survival depends on trying to predict its neuroticism in advance, sometimes using it as a partner to help fight the fire, all while they try to perfect **Standard Firefighting Order #10: Fight fires aggressively, providing for all safety first.**

Firefighters like Dan Steffensen understood this. He had trained countless hours to prevent the loss of wilderness, property, people, and his brotherhood. But as experienced as he was, there was no way he could have predicted or been mentally prepared for the summer of 2021.

A month before that dreadful season, he was sweeping the garage of Red Lodge Fire Rescue, a few blocks up on the historic Broadway Street, without an inkling that his life would soon be drastically changed.

A resident walking up Third Street saw him through the large open hangar door and shouted hello, but Dan merely grunted back at him. At age sixty-five, Dan had the reputation of being a little surly and a man of few words. But no one minded because he was a kind man at heart, and he had more than earned the right to be in whatever mood struck him.

When most Montana men his age were only concerned with catching their next Yellowstone cutthroat trout, Dan joined Red Lodge Fire

Rescue in 2016. He began a new career as a volunteer in his sixties and became a member of the familial firehouse that many town folks considered their second home.

Most of his friends described him with one word: tough. Dan was much like the land where he was born and chose to return to in the early 2000s. Living in Montana is hard-fought. Scenic grandeur invites a desire for permanence from tourists or those who dream of living in a movie. But temperatures below negative thirty degrees and snows six feet deep weary even the homegrown residents. During fire season, every sour smell of smoke or hazy-filled sky keeps neighbors and first responders on high alert. That's how Dan stayed. Alert.

The tall, lanky man was physically capable, and you knew you had his attention when he looked at you with his intense brown eyes over the thick mustache that he considered his rite of passage to fight fires. He started late in life, but firefighting consumed him, and he put everything he had into years of training to help battle the infamous Montana wildland fires.

His brow furrowed deeper. Dan swept around the various white vehicles, all marked with the large Red Lodge Fire Rescue logo in bold red. The engines were marked E78 and E77. An ambulance was marked A72 in the same bright red. A tender, or water truck, was T71.

Dan pushed the broomstick around with more gusto than was probably required for such a simple task. But it helped him work through the anger. Marney, his biggest supporter and the person who had his back while he chased his dreams, had died just a year prior. He was still furious that they hadn't let him see her in the hospital even though her illness had been unrelated to COVID. All the masks, vaccines, and policies in place now reminded him that he couldn't be with Marney when she most needed him. Because of this feeling of helplessness, he blamed himself for her suffering and ultimate death.

Dan continued sweeping, growling under his breath, all around the garage, from the big doors on Third Street to similarly large ones that opened on Broadway. There was a lot of space to sweep, but it was not enough for Dan. The anger didn't solve anything, but it gave him a kind of adrenaline that kept him from falling back into the dark emptiness he experienced after her death. It felt better to be angry than on the brink of despair.

Chief Tom Kuntz walked down the few steps from the firehouse into the garage and smiled sadly. He knew why Dan was so aggressive with his sweeping. But Chief Kuntz (Tom) also knew the man did not appreciate heart-to-heart talks. When Dan thought he was right about something, there was no arguing with him. His colleagues thought he was experiencing "Grumpy Old Man" syndrome—something firefighters acknowledged about themselves between fires—compounded for Dan by the loss of Marney.

"How's it going, Dan?" Tom asked. Tom was clean-cut, slim, and physically fit, but his hair often looked like he combed it with his fingers.

"Slow. It's a quiet day," Dan murmured.

"I'm grateful for that. Makes for a long day, but a safe and uneventful one." An awkward silence followed. Tom knew Dan was replacing Marney with Red Lodge Fire Rescue. "Hey, I just wanted to let you know how much I appreciate the time you spend here and with the recruits," said Tom.

Dan mumbled a thank you to the chief, who volunteered a quarter of his time to Red Lodge Fire Rescue. The nationally respected fire chief also owns the historic Pollard Hotel, Red Lodge Pizza Co., and other restaurants dotted between art galleries, antique shops, a coffee shop, a bakery, and a candy store. These establishments rest in the town known for its restored history of brick-faced walls and tin-squared ceilings.

Tom walked over to the open garage door and looked towards his town, just waking up at the base of Mount Maurice. He could almost smell the coffee house a block away. He knew a quiet day wouldn't last. The town knew it, too. Every Red Lodge citizen lived in a state of readiness to fight or evacuate. They were as keen as the local wildlife, able to react when they sensed danger from miles away. A woman sitting on her porch tensed when the petals on her flowers shook from the wind. An electrician working the line tightened his belt if the trees around him swayed.

Every resident heightens their senses, many digging in to defend their homes and livelihoods in the event of a disaster. A restaurant employee who teaches snowboarding volunteers for Red Lodge Fire Rescue. A local lawyer qualified in planning and operations on national wildland fires volunteers as a captain at Red Lodge Fire Rescue. A favorite elementary school teacher volunteers as a Red Lodge Fire Rescue firefighter. The camaraderie between Red Lodge Fire Rescue and the community not only overlaps—it multiplies.

When a six-foot-deep spring snow completely buries the town, a building roof collapses, or the Yellowstone River floods and washes out most of southeast Montana, the leadership of Red Lodge Fire Rescue doesn't flinch. Volunteers show up without being paged. Neighbors rescue neighbors.

It's as if the chief planned it that way. For decades, he has recruited and assembled a highly qualified family of shared respect. Tom walks down Broadway, stopping to meet everyone, shaking their hand, and making them feel like he is their brother or best friend. In his mind, each person he meets is a new Red Lodge Fire Rescue volunteer. Or they are the next friend needing to be rescued. Either way, they are part of his town, his extended family.

"Just another beautiful day out there!" shouted Captain Tyler Rae, walking into the garage. "The floor looks spotless!"

Tom gave him a look and tilted his head towards Dan, who was putting the broom away. Captain Rae (Tyler) understood and changed the subject. "It's quiet today." He was a fifteen-year veteran firefighter originally from Butte, Montana, with a thick neck almost as wide as his head and hair that always seemed like he had just removed his helmet.

Except when fighting fires, Tyler wore shorts all year, no matter how cold the temperature was outside. He supervised Red Lodge Fire Rescue's fuel mitigation crew, was a Red Lodge Fire Rescue training captain, and went out on national fire assignments as a logistics planning section chief on incident management teams or as an engine boss or task force leader.

He understood his friend Dan's need to be in the firehouse, even if it was just to beat the broom against the floor. On many fire missions, Dan and "Cap" Tyler sat in their engine for hours discussing fires and how to put them out safely. Cap mumbled, and Dan always sat with his one good ear facing toward a quietly rough voice he could barely hear.

Both were avid readers; Norman Maclean's *Young Men and Fire* was their particular favorite. Fire and families were their conversation topics during endless hours of waiting for plans to come together or for fires to blow.

"I don't want to jinx things by saying it's a quiet day," said Tom, smiling. He and Tyler headed back into the firehouse to review weekly training schedules.

Dan got the sponges and soap, ready to give an engine a good bath. He drove E78 into the parking lot, stopped, and looked east toward the sun. It was almost wholly above the horizon. He knew he should appreciate this yellow ball hanging in pure blue skies, making his world smell fresh and alive. But he felt nothing. He missed Marney and their Bernese Mountain dog, Lani, whom he had sent to live with Marney's daughter, Mandy Peck. If Dan was to be available to go on national firefights, he didn't think it was fair to Lani to be alone without him for long periods.

The void in his heart was a rift that kept getting deeper. And so, he washed the engine. Dan stopped working momentarily, closing his eyes, remembering a photo of Amanda Marsh, widow of Granite Mountain Hotshot leader Eric Marsh, who died with eighteen other men in the 2013 Yarnell Hill Fire. Her face haunted him. "She had no hope. Her expression was empty, revealing a tormented loss."

Dan questioned if he was glad to be alive. He sustained himself by thinking of the faces of everyone who cared about him and would suffer if he were gone—especially his family and Red Lodge Fire Rescue. Dan thought of the men who had trained and mentored him and the men and women he had mentored. He thought of his daughter Hannah Langenbahn and all the rest of his family. Dan did not want to cause anyone to feel the same despair he saw expressed in the photo of Amanda Marsh.

If he were going to make it, it would be for them, not for himself.

Dan breathed deeply through his nose, held the wilderness in his lungs, and let it out slowly. He supposed he could get through one more day. He would wake up and put one foot on the floor to rise from bed as he watched the sun rise with him outside his bedroom window. He would keep coming to the firehouse. He would keep sweeping, cleaning, and training until the next fire to fight.

He leaned into E78 and put his hand on the fender. He found one more spot to shine. Then he looked up and saw his reflection in the cab window. Looking back at him was the same expression of despair he saw on Amanda Marsh.

He asked himself what was next.

CHAPTER TWO

"I am a firefighter."

As Dan finished polishing E78, he heard a car horn honk and tires rolling across the gravel of the parking lot. He looked over to see an athletic, statuesque blonde getting out of her black SUV and walking toward him.

"Hey, Dan! Is the new training schedule up?" asked Sarah Ewald, who is considered Red Lodge Fire Rescue's "Chief Mother" and is the director of the Red Lodge Fire Rescue Foundation. Besides being a firefighter, she also coaches the high school girls basketball team and is married to local pilot Bo Ewald, who annually flies over the Fourth of July Parade.

Like Tom, Sarah "is" Red Lodge. Mention her name, and every response is, "Of course, I know Sarah. She helped me with this." Or, "I don't know what we would have done had she not taken the lead." She was among the first women to join Red Lodge Fire Rescue as a firefighter, directly recruited by the chief while having dinner in one of his restaurants.

Dan stopped to greet Sarah, putting down his sponge, stepping towards her, and pointing to the stairs to the firehouse. "They're putting it together right now."

Sarah's natural response was to put her arms out wide and meet Dan with a hug. "And good morning." The sun was higher in the sky now. Both wore sunglasses, but each could still read the other's eyes behind the dark shades. Dan smiled for the first time that morning. He put both arms around her waist, intertwined his fingers, and lowered his chin to meet her shoulder. She lingered longer than he did. He was always the first to let go. Still, Sarah was one of the few people Dan hugged.

He was slow to raise his chin as he turned away from her and returned to work in the garage. Sarah fondly shook her head. She couldn't get more than a few words from him, but she was one of his greatest fans. Sarah believed Dan was a part of the fabric of Red Lodge Fire Rescue, always pitching in, ready to travel or drive any truck. He was always ready to train or mentor a rookie. As Sarah walked up the stairs to the station offices, she couldn't imagine what they would do without him. Dan was family.

Firefighters have two families. One is the family with whom they work, train, and risk their lives, knowing this job will eventually kill them—probably not on duty, but from cancer, heart disease, stress, or even suicide. The other is their "blood" family with whom they miss many "firsts," as Captain Layne Hilton calls them—first steps, first days of school, first dances. Firefighters usually spend holidays with their crew instead of at home.

"Firefighters and first responders become comfortable with their own mortality. But they are not comfortable with the mortality of anyone else, especially their families," says Captain Hilton (Layne), Health and Wellness Officer for Salt Lake Unified Fire Authority.

It takes a unique type of person to be a member of this family. Tom told the *Billings Gazette* that "in an emergency situation it's not necessarily hard to find people to help, but that the greater challenge is finding people willing to be a part of an organization and train and be ready when they are needed over a period of time, even when it's a call in the middle of the night for people you don't know."

"That's something that Dan did," Tom told the *Gazette*.[1]

Dan had a reputation for being a dedicated firefighter. He had mastered tenders, trucks, engines, and breathing apparatuses. Beyond volunteering, he invested in a helmet light, gloves that worked best in structure fires, a radio harness essential for wildland fires, and everything else needed for added safety.

In class, he studied fire behavior by listening to Captain Will Bernard and analyzing the many posters on the station walls depicting how fuel (trees and grass) burns. Dan learned that grass fires move faster than forest fires and burn differently based on grass height, type, and moisture content. Forests have a high dead-to-live ratio with bug kill or frost, and trees can fall quickly, killing more firefighters than burnovers.

Still, the only way to truly learn fire behavior is to experience it and watch it become an uncontrollable animal that only cares about fuel and the speed and direction of the wind. The animal will climb a ridge, jump a canyon, and fly over a river or highway. It moans and howls louder than an oncoming tornado. Meeting this beast is the best incentive to train and train even more.

The inherent conflict of Order #10, achieving both safety for all and aggressive firefighting simultaneously, challenges all firefighters to find solace in failure. A wildland fire has a mercurial personality that is usually impossible to predict, even with well-trained technicians helping to determine the attack plan.

These technicians were Dan's family, fighting wildland fires and training him in the middle of a blast furnace. These men and women wore faces he never wanted to see sad or suffering. They were the people for whom he now lived. And whether he understood it or not, they felt the same for him.

As Sarah returned from the firehouse, she ran into Captain Bernard (Will), a tall yet stout bald man who looked like he could win a log-throwing contest. He was an attorney who graduated from the University of North Carolina at Chapel Hill, as everyone knew from the UNC sticker on each of his personal vehicles.

"Hey Sarah, how's everything? Nice day."

"It is, Will! I love spring."

"Enjoy it while you can and before we get any fires." Before he headed up the back stairs to his office, he turned to guide Dan, who was backing E78 into the garage. Will had spent the most time with Dan's formal training at the firehouse and is one of the most qualified and top trainers at Red Lodge Fire Rescue. Like Tyler, he goes out on national wildland fire assignments an average of over one hundred days each year as a planning section chief on incident management teams or as a task force leader.

Will is the same age as Dan but joined the structure fire service in Northern Virginia at age sixteen and has fourteen years of wildland fire experience. He is that guy that everyone goes to in a crisis. He is a professional firefighter known for bringing honor to Red Lodge Fire Rescue. If you have a question on policy, ask this captain. He gets everything right. He knows the history of professional firefighting and the organization.

As he watched Dan prepare to clean another vehicle, he thought about one of the many fires they had been on together.

The Thomas Fire

In December 2017, Montana sent two engine task forces and one engine strike team to the Thomas Fire in California.[2] One task force consisted of five wildland engines from western Montana and one wildland engine from Red Lodge Fire Rescue. Dan was one of the three-member Red Lodge Fire Rescue engine crew on Montana Task Force 5-6 led by Captain Bernard.

The strike team was designated Montana Strike Team 6 and was led by Captain Rae. It boasted five wildland engines from central Montana. Red Lodge Firefighter Hank Rae, Tyler's son, was engine boss on Engine 77 at Red Lodge Fire Rescue, with Dan as a crew member. Every engine boss has a favorite vehicle. Call it a fondness or a superstition. The engine boss sits in the passenger seat, often keeping their favorite snacks in the glove box of "their" engine. Hank is loyal to Engine 77 and mimics his father in wearing shorts but is skinny and able to walk incredible distances. Hank was the top dog in the required firefighter Pack Test: a hike of three miles in forty-five minutes with a forty-five-pound pack.

During the Thomas Fire, extreme Santa Ana turned the fire into a volcano-like force. Early in December, 1,000 firefighters fought the fire but achieved no containment. The fire consumed Grant Park above City Hall. Additional National Guard helicopters, Military C-130 airplanes, and hundreds of fire engines from Montana, and other western states had arrived to aid in the efforts.

Montana Task Force 5-6 and Strike Team 6 arrived at the Thomas Fire's Incident Command Post (ICP) at the Ventura County fairgrounds around December 8. They remained in Ventura for two days, watching the fire over the hill blow bigger and waiting for their assignments, firefighters pressed black tape onto their trucks in mourning following the death of Corey Iverson.

In Matthew Desmond's book *On the Fireline*, he recalls how firefighters react to the death of a friend. "My crewmembers did not pose any new questions at the time . . . because the only questions that mattered to them had already been asked (and answered) a few days after he was burned: What did he do wrong? What should he have done differently? These questions, though they can take many forms, are but one question—the question of fault—and it haunts all who demand to know why wildland firefighters get caught up in deadly situations."[3]

This is why they always tried to solve the puzzle before they faced the beast. Task Force 5-6 laid thousands of feet of hose and cut fire breaks late into their twenty-four-hour shifts, thinking they could defend the homes below the Tea Garden in Montecito. The plan was to wait for the fire to come out of the rugged backcountry into more favorable terrain where firefighters could attack the fire safely. The morning the fire finally crested the hill and raged into Montecito, it became a battle to triage and save as many homes as possible. The hose lays were meaningless. The fire wiped them out as if they were paper straws.

These were hard lessons for firefighters. No matter how many hours they dedicated to a plan of attack, it often failed in a flash. And instead of letting the failure forever bruise their egos, they had to regroup and keep fighting. On this fire, as with many, the best-laid plans fell victim to extreme conditions created by uncontrollable winds.

Finally, the winds weakened, allowing firefighters to contain the fire. On December 21, Santa Barbara County lifted evacuation orders. The Montana firefighters returned home on December 23.

Home to Family

Although they were often considered firefighters first and spouses or parents second, the team was glad to return to their families. That year, Dan went home to Marney. They proved the adage "opposites attract." While he stood over six feet tall, she barely topped five feet. While she was polished and professional, he was rough, using a cuss word in every other sentence.

"They were an acutely odd couple," says Sarah. "She had her nails done every week. Firefighting was out of her norm. But he loved it, and she loved him."

Together for over fifteen years, both had two adult children from previous marriages. Hannah Langenbahn and Will Steffensen, who live in Ohio and Missouri respectively, are Dan's children. Margot Dickinson and Mandy Peck are Marney's daughters; they are almost a decade older than Hannah and Will, and also live in Ohio. There were a few visits back and forth, but for the most part, it was just Dan, Marney, and Lani, their dog.

"Marney fed my need to satisfy my ego," says Dan. "She knew that was what made me go. After I sold my business, I wanted to be a fishing guide. A big push was from her. I wanted to do fire. 'Well, let's make that happen.' Marney was always my biggest supporter. If there was ever a time that she wanted me to stay home, she never said it. My ego probably wasn't listening. Or I didn't want to know."

Marney's daughter, Mandy, says, "It terrified her every time he left the house. She hated it. But she loved him."

Layne says most firefighters are afraid to ask if the life is too hard or frightening for their loved ones. If their family ever said, "I hate that you are a firefighter," it would be the same as saying, "I hate you." It's an I AM profession, not an I DO profession.

"I am a teacher."

"I am a doctor."

"I am a firefighter."

Dan is a firefighter. His passion and dedication came from an inner calling long before that fateful summer.

CHAPTER THREE

"This is where I need to be."

WHEN HE WAS SIX YEARS OLD, DAN SCARED HIS MOTHER AND SISTER, who came running out into the yard thinking he was in danger. But he had things under control; he was only shouting orders at his imaginary fire crew, pretending the garden was ablaze and drowning it with the garden hose. He imagined he was a fireman because his uncle, Les Corcoran, was the fire chief in Idaho Falls and would let him climb into the fire engines whenever Dan visited. His sister, Cindy Northey, reminisces how they always either played fireman or wagon train, using their big bunk beds for the appropriate mode of transportation. Dan can't remember not wanting to be a firefighter.

When he was fifteen, Dan read Dennis Smith's *Report from Engine Co. 82,* which describes brave men fighting big fires with rudimentary equipment and constant action. Dan loved how they stood beside and behind each other in impossible conditions. Heroism and camaraderie were involved in aggressively fighting structure fires. To do it well and live, you had to be alert, stay calm, think clearly, and act decisively. Dan used these same standards when building a fence or catching a fish. He related to the firefighters in the book, seemingly at their best in a crisis, men with egos needing to be fed with difficult tasks to perform. He was more drawn to them with every page, knowing he was just like them.

Firefighting tugged at Dan for most of his life. He succumbed to the pull when he and Marney returned to his Montana home. Although being with a firefighter was not an aspiration of her own, she encouraged him to follow his dream. He thought she supported him when she said, "I will take care of the dog and me."

One time, the Red Lodge Roman Theatre held a special showing of *Only the Brave* for firefighters and their families. As he left the movie, a colleague asked him, "Where's Marney?"

Dan said, "She didn't want to see this. It hits too close to home."

The friend commented, "You're only running a tender; what kind of trouble can you get into?"

Dan had been in a tight spot on the Lolo Peak fire but did not bother explaining that to his friend, who had never been on anything more than a one-acre fire. Still, the comment pissed Dan off. It was a challenge. He was resolved to be the best wildland firefighter he could be. Dan wanted to get on and face the big fires that would test his expertise and courage.

He had something to prove. He was motivated by the challenge and difficulty of the required skills. The bigger the challenge, the greater the motivation. No matter his age or the lifestyle of having to leave at a moment's notice. No matter how it affected his home and the person he left behind.

But in 2019, when COVID-19[1] was the underlying cause of over a million deaths in the United States, Marney was hospitalized for an illness that had nothing to do with the pandemic.

"They wouldn't let me in to see her. I argued with them to let me see her, and they wouldn't let me in," Dan says. He imagined her desperately deteriorating, crying for him, confused that he was not beside her, holding her hand. He felt impotent, helpless.

She was heavily medicated and unable to advocate for herself. When he felt sure she would have chosen to live, instead, according to Dan, she agreed to enter hospice care, possibly not realizing that once in, she was not coming out.

Like all first responders, Dan could not cope with feeling helpless. A first responder's purpose is to stop loss. But loss is inevitable, leaving them fighting a losing battle. Guilt, frustration, and even anger are thus part of the job. Dan crushed all of these emotions to their limits as Marney lay dying.

When she was sent home for hospice care, her pain was heinous. Her daughters, Mandy and Margot, were there to help make her as comfortable as possible. But for her final days, it would just be Dan. She never got out of bed. He lay beside her, holding her, even if she didn't know he was there. *He* knew.

The doctors only had one suggestion for him, which they offered daily. "'Give her more morphine,'" he says they told him. "I did. I gave her more morphine."

On Thursday, May 7, 2020, Marney died. Dan slowed his steps and stood with his arms hanging low. The side of his mouth and his eyes sagged. This emotional wound was more profound than any physical one he would ever endure.

Dan says, "I was her protector, and I didn't protect her. I killed her. And you will never be able to convince me otherwise."

Margot and Mandy disagree with him. They felt that Dan's care, for many years, helped Marney to live as long as she did. "If he has done anything well in his life, it was taking care of our mother," says Mandy. "But we were concerned then that he had given up."

That Saturday after Marney died, Dan was in the grip of an emptiness so deep there was nothing to keep him standing. He could feel himself collapsing, with only darkness ahead of him. Her death left an impossible and dismal void in his life. She was his everything. When something good happened, she was the first one he wanted to tell. There was only one place where he could erase the helplessness plaguing him: Red Lodge Fire Rescue. Dan still had his brothers and sisters on the fire line. They were all he had.

Dan walked to the back of the garage, where Will had parked a tender to conduct a nozzle training session for several recruits. Will saw Dan dressed for training in his boots and fireproof pants, coming around the corner of the big gray building. He asked the recruits to give him a minute, then met Dan and put his big, paw-like hands on Dan's shoulders.

"Dan, I just heard Marney died two days ago. Why are you here?"

Dan looked at Will blankly and glanced over his shoulder to the tender and the recruits with the nozzles in their hands. He said, "This is where I need to be."

Will, or "Cap" to Dan while on duty, had trained Dan in the classroom and the field for several years. As much as he wanted to give the firefighter a grizzly bear hug, man to man, he knew Dan would not want it in front of these young trainees.

Instead, Will pumped his fists against Dan's shoulders and thought about his first training with him. The captain always recognizes the behaviors of "go-getters" and "team players" when Red Lodge Fire Rescue recruits begin training. He often correctly guesses whether a recruit has a military background or has played competitive team sports or individual sports.

Dan had always played solo in accomplishing his goals in life—or, as he admits, in feeding his ego. He was a fly-fishing guide in Idaho and an exhibition skydiver in Kings Island with over 1,100 jumps. Finally, the pinnacle for him was firefighting, a team sport.

At one point, Will had to tell him, "Dan, training is not a competition." He wanted the recruit to stop training as a competitor against the other trainees. Dan needed experience on large fires to understand how the team functioned and his role as a member of a professional organization.

Dan said, "Everything I do is a competition." His fierce spirit usually paid off because he excelled at everything he tried. But he soon found out that no one was keeping score. Being the best was not important. He got disapproving comments, such as "does not play well with others." In his own words, he "did not suffer fools well."

He just wanted everyone to be safe. He lived by Order #10: fight aggressively but safely. There was always more to learn, practice, train, and mentor. That is what he loved. It was *all* he loved.

If Dan ever missed a detail, he would put his head down and quietly say, "Well fuck," to admonish himself and try harder. Everyone in his training classes had heard him utter those words, and they often chuckled, appreciating his self-deprecation and renewed dedication. They would have been even more impressed or perhaps empathetic if they had known about his physical condition. Dan had rheumatoid arthritis and dealt with a lot of pain in his joints; when it flared, he couldn't even move certain body parts. The flares and pain moved around to different joints.

Now that Marney and Lani were gone, Dan bought a new home within five minutes of the firehouse. He kept most of the furniture he shared with Marney. Every arm on every chair and sofa held a pillow she had needlepoint. Every flat surface held several framed photos of just her. His home was a shrine to Marney, except for the pictures of fires and firefighters.

He aligned every eventful decision with his commitment to Red Lodge Fire Rescue and traveling to big fires. He was taking control of what he saw as his only destiny: being the best firefighter he could be.

Fighting large wildland fires was where Dan and others learned the art of a safe fight—the importance of lookouts, communications, escape routes, and safety zones, and how to work with other agencies on the fire ground effectively. They watched how a fire moves and grows, always planning their escape route to a safe location. Every fire is a new classroom, with every backfire a new chapter and every exploding pine tree a period at the end of a sentence.

He fought fires in Colorado, Oregon, Wyoming, and California whenever the opportunity for help from Red Lodge Fire Rescue arose. He always brought home a T-shirt from the area firehouse. These fires were where he completed the task books and training necessary to become an engine boss.[2] And even though he didn't know it, because no one did, every moment of instruction and every chance for training would eventually lead to the biggest battle of his life.

The August Complex Fire

Having qualified as an engine boss, Dan earned his first opportunity to lead a wildland fire engine assigned to a major out-of-state fire incident. In the fall of 2020, Montana firefighters deployed to other states, including California. Red Lodge Fire Rescue sent a wildland engine to the August Complex, a group of thirty-eight fires started by lightning strikes on August 16 and 17 in the Coast Range of Northern California. The fires were focused in the Six Rivers National Forest and the Mendocino National Forest.

Dan and his crew on the Red Lodge Fire Rescue engine arrived at the August Complex on September 4. A whirlwind of fire activity in eastern Mendocino County led to an evacuation warning for the Mendocino National Forest. On September 5, the National Weather

Service issued a Fire Weather Warning due to high winds and unseasonably hot temperatures of 90 to 110 degrees Fahrenheit.[3]

The August Complex was deep in the bowels of the forest, so to enter this devil's playground, they had to cut down trees. The weather was warm, even hot, with a small amount of wind, creating a unique and almost impossible situation to work with. Smoke was not escaping because of a persistent inversion, wiping out any chance for air support.

Dan's division's Incident Action Plan (IAP) assignment was to construct a fuel break or light a backfire to stall the fire's growth. He and his engine crew could see the fire ten miles away as they confirmed radio frequencies. Their escape route was a "long, twisty, crappy road, steep places but not too steep." Along the road they set vehicles in place as "trigger points"— predetermined spots as prompts for firefighters to potentially reevaluate the plan if the fire behavior or weather changes. Depending on time and distance to safety, trigger points can quickly turn into what Tyler calls "oh crap" points, where they are losing control and have to give it up.

Safety zones were downslope and upwind. They started a backfire, often using drip torches at anchor points such as a road or river to consume the fuel in the path of the oncoming wildfire. In this case, they used a half-mile of hose lays. Every two hundred feet, they connected another hose for another firefighter to manage.

Everything was fine until the hose blew at Dan's engine. They shut everything down, left their hose, and departed in their engine. It was late in the day and soon it would be too dark for a lookout.[4]

Although they already had a crappy escape route, command suggested that they try to stop the fire from spreading at the road by backfiring along the natural road. But deep down, Dan knew it was a long shot. Without a lookout, they lost the fire overnight.

The next morning's briefing at the Incident Command Post (ICP) reviewed the weather and the fire behavior. They decided to focus on structure protection, and the crew began preparing a dozen houses in that area for the fire.

One home captured the team's heart because a United States of America flag was flying over it. It looked like the home was defendable, so they removed propane tanks, gas tanks, and spray cans. At first, Dan wanted to stay with the structure. But he was his own lookout. He saw a spot fire one hundred yards away. Their escape was back from where they came. There were also half a dozen outbuildings that he knew they could not save.

He called the Incident Commander (IC)[5] on the radio. "Command, we gotta go." Dan was always a man of few words. Two to four syllables often said everything. Most of his communication was in his eyes. Sometimes, they were angry, looking out from under his brows with his chin pointed down. This time, they were straight-on determined.

Dan cut down the flag that was still flying above the house. He carried it with them on their way out. Three days later, they went back to the home. It was all gone.

They returned the saved flag to the homeowner. Still, Dan felt the loss as deeply as if it had been his own pile of burned treasure.

It took Dan a long time to get over the loss of that home. Dan says, "It's someone's everything. That is someone's sanctuary, someone's refuge. It is full of all the things that define who we are. Pictures. Knick-knacks. Toys for the kids or grandkids. Stuff. Yeah, it's only stuff, but it's their stuff. They count on firefighters to save that home and their stuff. And we have taken an oath to do everything we can to save it. Losing that one hurt."

The home was part of the inevitable loss firefighters live with. According to Layne, first responders must find meaning in loss to keep the psychological and spiritual losses from piling up.

Dan's engine crew stayed on the August Complex until September 21. On September 24, due to the success of back-burning, the fire held south of State Route 36, allowing Montana firefighters to return home.

Nothing to Risk

When Dan returned home alone, he was aching to feel something. It had been months since Marney died. Through pictures and needlepoint, Marney was everywhere in his house. But *she* wasn't there. He was living with, loving, a ghost. He seemed to have nothing to lose or win and, therefore, nothing to risk.

Erving Goffman first articulated the concept "To risk is to be a man" in his essay "Where the Action Is," over fifty years ago. Goffman's argument was based on the relationship between action and *character*. "The voluntary taking of serious chances is a means for *the maintenance and acquisition of character*."[6]

In his book *On the Fireline*, Matthew Desmond considered Goffman's theory when he wrote, "Firefighting—marching, digging, chopping, crawling, and running among torching trees and smoldering ash—is a corporeal activity, and in the swelter of infernos, firefighters' bodies react to the dangers they face. *How far should I go down the canyon wall? How much heat can I take? Is this dangerous, or am I scared? Is that oak burned straight through? Is that smoke or steam? Should I keep digging, or should I fall back?*"[7]

Ironically, when these firefighters are not risking death, they risk depression, coping with binge drinking, or eventual divorce.[8] The end of a fire season, though very good for the affected people, is not good for firefighters, going from long days battling a fire, saving a town or a home, to returning to a normal life.

Dan quotes Jimmy Buffet's "The Captain and the Kid": "His world had gone from sailing ships to raking mom's backyard / He never could adjust to land, although he tried so hard." Without Marney and Lani,

Dan was especially susceptible to a loss of purpose. For him and his ego, now, it was hard to be a man or maintain character without something to risk. The other ingredient, the woman in his life, was also gone.

Dan had given up the Mormon religion in which he was raised. And he is an alcoholic who gave up drinking twenty years ago. The idea of leaning on a higher power had been drilled into him early and then reinforced. He also understood the concept of taking inventory of his life. Coping skills were intrinsic to his character in dealing with grief and loneliness. Now, he had a new dependency: firefighting and Red Lodge Fire Rescue. Fire was his new addiction. When not fighting them, he was training for them.

As Layne would soon come to understand, Red Lodge is bonded across firefighter and blood families in a way he had never witnessed anywhere else in the world. Tom, Tyler, Will, Sarah, and others went out of their way to care for Dan, to fill his emotional hole where they could, so much so that the people of Red Lodge became the blanket that tucked him in bed at night. They didn't realize they were in training to face the tragedy-riddled sixty-nine days in the coming summer.

Everyone, from the pastor to the poet, would soon live with a sense of mortality that was a car parked on the main street of town, needing to be towed away. Every citizen, firefighter, Emergency Medical Technician (EMT), and rescuer would come through as if God had commanded them to give each other their greatest skills, courage, and love.

CHAPTER FOUR

Fire Season Came Early

Rookie firefighter Katy Hedtke was on her way home from a quick stop to buy milk at the Beartooth IGA just off Broadway, a couple blocks from the firehouse. She was on summer break from teaching her elementary students. As a volunteer firefighter and EMT, she found that keeping staples such as milk at home was often neglected until the last moment.

In her late twenties and standing at 5'4", she wore her long blonde hair in braids and smiled at another customer as if she were everyone's best friend, even though she didn't recognize them. This was one of the few times her fresh, cream-colored face wasn't dirty with fire ash proudly worn after working in the field. Able to keep up with any man on the mountain, fighting fires or hunting elk, Katy would be easily mistaken for one of the guys except for her close, devoted pack of girl pals.

It was June. She had just driven over a two-mile bridge when she looked at her watch. It read 13:13 when the page came from her cell phone. It was an alert from the Carbon County Sheriff's Office that smoke had been seen rising six miles south of Mount Maurice. Katy turned her truck around. Within three minutes, she was at the firehouse, leaving the freshly purchased milk for her husband to retrieve later. She changed into her wildland fire gear, joining Dan and firefighter Brad Milligan in Engine 78. Captain Mark Koter drove a tender. Just as Hank was loyal to Engine 77, Dan claimed Engine 78 as his. The engines were not assigned to any specific firefighter, but Dan rode in the passenger seat as engine boss and kept his Mentos in the glove box.

The tender and the engine pulled out of the fire station, racing to catch up with Chief Kuntz, sirens blaring, starting the neighborhood dogs howling. Captain Koter (Mark), driving the tender filled to the top with water, could feel Broadway vibrate beneath him. They were heading south for what they knew was the terrain of canyons and dense forest beyond the rambling hills of sage and dry grass.

Both vehicles turned on Highway 308, which led to the tiny towns of Belfry and Bear Creek, and then south on Highway 72 towards the Wyoming border to meet up with the chief, where he had stopped to stage for the fight. A spiral of smoke was growing from a draw to the west. Many draws led to canyons that crawled up the south side of Mount Maurice. Brad stayed with the tender, and Katy and Captain Koter jumped in Engine 78 with Dan to drive closer to see the fire. They left the pavement and bounced onto the gravel road, kicking up dust through the open fields.

An engine and a water tender crew from another town's fire department had also heard the call and responded, staying very close to the Red Lodge crew.

Katy, Captain Koter, and Dan stayed on high ground opposite the fire on the Robertson Draw Road. From that vantage point, they could see the fire wasn't moving, benign, almost hiding, stuck in the draw with the possibility of heading away from them, north and up towards a high ridge. The weather was barely conducive for fire, with no wind to encourage it at that point. They had no resources except for themselves, so Dan tried to call for a spot weather check.

He looked down at the fire, frowning and looking carefully for signs of potential erratic fire behavior. They all knew the beast was moody and capable of causing suffering, destruction, and even death.

Fighting fires in Red Lodge[1] is typical for Montana. This state has large, fast-moving fires caused by high winds and dry fuels, sometimes naturally started by lightning, other times by man. Forest Service and Bureau of Land Management (BLM) lands buttress Red Lodge, with the Beartooth Mountains and Custer National Forest forming the impeding hand of God, telling them this is as far as the city can go. Nature takes it from here.

These fires move quickly and are difficult to suppress in timber and grass. North of the town are miles of open grassland and cattle ranches supported by small towns, including Roberts and Joliet, all within Carbon County, which has a population of 10,000. The city of Red Lodge, the county seat, is the largest, with a population of 2,200. The grasslands finally meet the Yellowstone River sixty miles north, heading east to the confluence of the Missouri River in North Dakota.

"Hey! What are they doing?" shouted Katy. They saw the other town's engine crew trying to drive up the draw opposite their position, full of dead grass, sage, down trees, and unburned fuel. All three Red Lodge crew members yelled, "Don't go up there! It's too steep!"

That engine crew seemed to be in the throes of a God complex. The IRPG[2] identifies seven Hazardous Attitudes, which include thinking one is "Invulnerable" and just being too damn "Macho." Sometimes, an engine or truck crew unreasonably believes they can take a vehicle up a steep and rocky slope to check out a fire. And engaging in mob mentality is extremely dangerous in this line of work. "Group Think," or being afraid to speak up or disagree, is also one of the listed Hazardous Attitudes. Dan was never scared to voice his opinions, especially about incompetence, perceived or actual. Nor was Katy.

The engine crew ignored their warning, went in, and got a flat tire. The Red Lodge firefighters shook their heads, unable to help from their position on the Robertson Draw road.

They could see the black[3]—the area where the fire had already burned and was considered a safe zone. The trail leading into the draw had stopped the fire, leaving the black butting next to it on one side, the other still unburnt.

"I think I can walk in there safely," Dan told the captain.

"Okay, be careful. Keep us in the loop."

"I'll take a radio. Katy, do you want to go with me?" Dan had been Katy's mentor through much of her training. Besides having a "nose" for fire, she knew the area well because she hunted for shed antlers there.

"I'm down," she said.

They followed the trail where the black opened up more. Without wind, the fire was as quiet as a ghost, which could be as terrifying as the loud jet engine sound of roaring flames. At that point, they couldn't see any flames, only smoke. But Dan knew it was going up the draw, where a ton of unburned fuel would hit the ridge's end.

At the foot of the draw, two men stopped them and told them a man on a motorcycle started the fire. Up the trail, Dan and Katy were surprised to find this man, John Lightburn, still on the trail, kneeling by his bike and looking sheepish. He had been trying to escape before getting caught, hoping the firefighters didn't see him.

"Stay with the radio," Dan told Katy. He didn't know if the man was dangerous, so he wanted to check the guy out.

"I tried to replace a spark plug," the man explained. "I think I poked a fuel line. I'm so sorry! It was an accident. I didn't mean to start a fire!"

Dan signaled for Katy to come over.

"Hey, are you okay?" asked Katy, who noticed he was unsteady on his feet, even though he was trying to leave. She saw he was burned on his chest and feet. "I'm an EMT. I can help," she said.

"I just want to get out of here." He tried to take off, but they talked him into staying with them. Then they radioed for a side-by-side to meet them at the trailhead as they escorted him back out to be arrested.[4] Katy turned him over to EMTs waiting on the road so she could stay with the firefighting crew.

"I'm here to fight the fire," she said. Katy grabbed Dan's arm to ensure everyone knew she was with him and headed out again. It was important to her because this was her first real wildland fire.

They continued to follow the trail next to the black, calling for air support on the way and developing a plan for water drops. Dan and Katy climbed the hill above the gulch to direct the helicopter. He could see a thunderstorm rambling in, which he hoped would help put the fire out. But he could not get a spot weather report in that location because the terrain blocked his phone signal. The National Weather Service (NWS) in Billings for Yellowstone County often took twenty minutes to respond with updates.

Dan radioed back to Chief Kuntz, still positioned on Highway 72 and unable to see anything, but Dan could now see the fire had gone around the corner from the black, deep into the draw. It was sending flames high enough that embers were starting to float down on their position.

"Do you know how to direct water drops?" the chief asked.

"I got this."

Dan directed the helicopter for drops to protect their position and control spot fires. Then, with a tanker coming in, he transferred the helicopter water drops to Katy so that he could direct the tanker drop of retardant.

It was also Katy's first drop.

"Follow your IRPG. You've got this," Dan told her.

She opened the IRPG: "Identify any flight hazards, finalize the location with clock positions from the pilots' location, describe prominent landmarks, and convey the target position on the slope—lower 1/3, upper 1/3, mid-slope, or top of the ridge."[5] She radioed the pilots to start dropping water on an active fire.

Although Dan had never guided an air tanker, he had listened to hundreds of hours of others doing it. He was confident he could do it safely. When he said, "Well fuck," that meant he had more to learn. But everyone knew Dan was in control when he said, "I got this."

He directed the tanker retardant drop on a practice line, downhill into the wind and away from the sun. He could hear the engine before he saw its wingspan soaring like a golden eagle approaching a river or expansive pasture seeking its next meal. This colossal bird sought the perfect line in which to blanket the bright red retardant. But this was a practice run. The tanker lifted gracefully, without its prey, banked its full body to the right, and circled.

"Is that where you want it?" the pilot asked Dan.

"That would be perfect," he said.

The roar of the tanker engines came back as they followed the same line for the retardant drop. Dan watched as the metal bird glistened and delivered what seemed like a thick, never-ending waterfall right where he wanted it. And as if it had captured its prey, the bird pulled up into the sky and was gone as soon as it had come.

Both Katy and Dan directed the air drops perfectly.

Dan would remember that experience with appreciation. "When an aircraft goes by at 150 miles per hour at your level, and you can see the pilot has Ray Ban sunglasses on, it is a rush no one else can ever know or describe."

That day, that fire, Dan realized he could trust himself. He had a sense of quiet confidence. He knew he was a good firefighter and the best he could be. After California, Colorado, Wyoming, and Oregon and hours of training, he had the opportunity to fight the fire near his hometown, which was personally significant to him. Dan took charge of assigned resources, assessed the situation by gaining intel, took the initiative in the absence of others, communicated specific instructions, and even supervised at the scene. He could see how the fire behaved as he utilized resources and kept track of an ever-changing situation. It came together to give him a sense of peace and strength in his ability to be a vital team member and a leader. His relationship with firefighting was finally filling the chasm from the loss of Marney.

Dan and Katy were getting a line, or moving fuel from the edge of the fire so that it would no longer burn, with hand tools around in a circle on the west side. They wanted to stay and watch the fire all night, but they were ordered out because of reported grizzly bears in the area. They slept in the engine and left a Type 5 fire behind them, small with little complexity and almost under control.

Arriving back on the scene the morning of the 14th, the fire was now a Type 4, considered an incident requiring an IC, heading north and into the forest up the back of Mount Maurice. By 6:30 p.m. on June 15, the fire had traveled six miles, slopping over the top of Mount Maurice like a spooked herd of elk, desperate to trample Red Lodge. The body of the beast was mainly on Forest Service land and very difficult to access.

As it fed on more fuel, it expanded to bigger fire types. Every day, firefighters were required to start over with new management and communications. Every time the fire type changed, so did command. The plan of attack and levels of bureaucracy changed with them. When the local Forest Service District Office set up a Type 3 incident management team, Captain Rae was assigned to oversee logistics. The Forest Service could have gone to him directly for resources. Instead, they went to the federal government, then to the state, and finally to

Captain Rae, who was on site. Thus, resources were delayed by a day because of unnecessary lines of communication.

The incident management team brought in Red Lodge Fire Rescue Deputy Chief Tim Ryan, a tall, slim man who always dipped his lip on the right when he smiled. He was a talented chef who took over ownership of the Bear Creek Saloon in neighboring Bear Creek when the prior owner passed away. While Chief Ryan (Tim) handled finances and the North Division of the fire, Chief Kuntz was in charge of the East Division.

Captain Bernard took charge of planning for the Robertson Draw Fire. Red Lodge Assistant Chief Jon Trapp was assigned to operations, including establishing contact with a meteorologist[6] for real-time weather spot checks. Assistant Chief Trapp (Jon), an eleven-year fire veteran, also worked full-time for Red Lodge Fire Rescue. Tall and fit, he is a bit baby-faced, though in his forties. His stature is that of an officer in the Air Force, yet in his heart, he is a mountain man. He is an expert tracker, wolf biologist, and fire behaviorist, always going out of his way to explain different terrain and weather behavior. As a national wind, fuel, and fire behavior consultant, he is the guy who finds the images and posters to pin to the walls.

While management was being implemented for the Robertson Draw Fire, the residents of Red Lodge watched the flames and smoke devour Mount Maurice. The moment of disaster they all dreaded was at their feet, with only their courage to stop it.

"The day the fire came over that hill was as chaotic as any I have seen," recalls Dan. "And it was my backyard, a reality I had never faced before."

That night, Dan got home to sleep in his bed. At four in the morning, Captain Rae, in charge of resources for what was now a Type 2 fire, woke him up and said, "Get back here with a tender."

A second fire erupted just to the east: the Crooked Creek Fire. Dan was assigned to take the tender there on June 22. The fire was near the Ice Caves in the Pryor Mountains. They were known for being the home of wild mustangs, protected on BLM land. These magnificent animals often kept Dan company as he operated the tender until the 27th.

One of the people hearing the sirens leaving town that first day of the Robertson Draw Fire was Ruth Bilyeu, director of community care[7] and an advanced EMT for Red Lodge Fire Rescue. She knew it was her firefighters responding to the call. She anxiously looked out the window of the firehouse, hoping for their return. Whenever that happened, her firefighters would jump out of the engines and guide the driver safely back through the tall doors into the garage, another job well done.

Not this time; she watched in anguish as seventy-two hours later, Mount Maurice became an inferno, turning at its base like a tornado picking up speed. Red and yellow flames at the bottom of the spiral caused a tower of smoke to spin higher and wider.

Her mind went to the Willie Fire of 2000, named for a Willie Nelson concert that was in progress at the time. "I was trying to remember everything we learned from that fire. We had evacuated the nursing home patients and some homes going up Bear Creek. A motorcycle crash started it. I thought it was all hands on deck. Dozer lines saved the city, then."

Ruth is tall with a determined face that reflects her twenty-three years as an EMT and growing up as a downhill skier in Wyoming. Red Lodge ski mountain is her mountain. She and Sarah are each other's person. The bond of trust is not only observable; it can be felt sitting across a firehouse room that is sometimes an office and sometimes a dormitory. They get through any crisis or trauma in the Red Lodge

Fire Rescue family together, taking charge of the station and leaning on each other by sharing the hard truth of their drowning emotions.

The Willie Fire was one such instance when everyone came together. "The station was hectic as we made more beds available for firefighters. People kept donating things. We started spreading the word to bring food and water. People wanted to help. They needed to feel like they contributed to in a crisis," says Ruth.

That was twenty years ago, and it was scary enough then. Looking out the window, the flames of this Robertson Draw Fire were growing hotter and running fast at her town. Smoke billowed beyond the reach of eyesight. The intense smell made her wonder if God was angry with the valley.

Her only comfort was knowing firefighters now had many more resources than in 2000 and improved abilities to watch and predict fire behavior. The twirling nature of the fire meant it was picking up speed. All her engines were braced between the fire and the town, just waiting for it to come down from the forest into the grassy fuel where they could beat it down. Every available Red Lodge Fire Rescue member was involved in some aspect of the fire.

Then, as if a mighty hand reached down and bent it around the mountain, the wind shifted away from the town. The fire headed east, where approximately 2,500 structures were in the path of what became a runaway train tearing up the Beartooth Canyon. Engines had come from all over the state waiting in its path, assigned positions to push the fire back into the wilderness, away from humanity.

Ruth kept the station ready to handle the crush of people arriving for the battle. Offices became dormitories. Coolers filled up with bottled water.

Finally, the Forest Service took over, and the fire management was moved to Belfry, where the fire had now decided to live. Over the next two weeks, more outside resources relieved Dan and Katy and another rookie, firefighter Scott Wilson, so that they could focus on the local region.

Like Dan, Scott had retired and became a firefighter late in life. Married with children and grandchildren, he seemed innocent with his clean face and quiet demeanor but was committed and eager to learn. Dan mentored Katy and Scott while the chiefs and captains were all sucked into the Robertson Draw incident management team over Forest Service and BLM firefighters.

When the Forest Service assumed leadership of the Robertson Draw incident management team, Captain Bernard was called to Alaska to assist with another fire. He and Captain Rae were members of the Northern Rocky Team 6, a Type 2 incident management team, as the planning and logistics section chiefs, respectively. Both would often be called to other national fires and away from Red Lodge. Deputy Chief Ryan wasn't released from the Robertson Draw Fire until the first snows in November.

The Robertson Draw Fire became like a visiting cousin sleeping in the guest room. It was mostly contained, with a constant presence of smoke on the southern horizon of the Beartooths, but would eventually burn over 30,000 acres. The heavy fuel on the edge of town had burned to completion.

Everyone prepared for the annual Fourth of July weekend celebration. The ongoing wilderness fire containment that would continue until November did not deter the rush of tourists, who annually increase the population tenfold for the parade and Rodeo of Champions, culminating with fireworks. Every restaurant and hotel is booked in advance for months.

KTVQ news said, "Even with two wildfires and Stage II fire restrictions starting Friday, people are ready to celebrate Independence Day in Red Lodge. Fire crews continue to work on the Robertson Draw Fire south of Red Lodge, which is at 65 percent containment."

Carbon County Commissioner Bill Bullock reassured residents that it was safe to celebrate the holiday. "There's some hotspots, but they're paying very close attention to them," he told KTVQ News. "They still got some aircraft here for support and water drops and retardant drops. They're prepped for anything that comes up."[8]

A more false statement could not have been made that day. The days from June 13 to August 21 were marked by four catastrophes. The Robertson Draw Fire was the first. The sum of all four would result in this period being christened "The Summer of Hell."

CHAPTER FIVE

"Severity is painful."

FIREWORKS HAD BLASTED INTO THE SKY, BLOCKING OUT THE STARS for an hour on the night of July 4th. Then, fire engines were all tucked into the station garage, asleep, grateful for no calls for the holiday. But the quiet mood would disintegrate into a frenzy the following day.

Dan, who had been relieved from the Crooked Creek Fire, and Katy, both frustrated not to be fighting fires, had been cutting down trees on fuel crew duty, which is typical while on severity.[1] It was physically grueling work, so much so that Dan had worn out his firefighting gloves and was, at the time, wearing leather gloves on wildland fires.

"Help! Help! She's missing!"

They looked up from the station's cement garage floor where they were cleaning their saws to see Tatum Morrell's mother in tears. She was frantic yet fierce, terrified that her daughter was in trouble. Pacing around the garage, arms flailing seemed to be the only thing she could do, for when she stopped and stood still, her body trembled violently.

"What's wrong? What happened?" asked Katy, who stood up and tried to comfort her.

"Tate! She went hiking, and she hasn't come back! I haven't heard from her in days!"

Dan recognized the pain of loss on the woman's face. It was the same as the reflection in his mirror when he lost Marney.

"We will help you," said Dan as he stood up and reached out with an empathetic hand.

Tatum, an athletic twenty-three-year-old and avid hiker, had just graduated from Montana State University in Bozeman and was exploring the Beartooth Mountains before starting a new job as an engineer in Bozeman. Taking such trips wasn't unusual for her, but she was always safety conscious and routinely checked in with her family.

"Hey, Jon is here today," said Katy, running to get him out of the office. The assistant chief, who was in charge of full-time Search and Rescue (SAR), got to work right away for the missing hiker, ready to take on double duty. He was still assisting with operations for the Robertson Draw Fire.

"What can I do to help?" Lieutenant Amy Hyfield asked, walking into the station. The 5'4" firefighter, SAR member, and EMT doesn't take no for an answer, except maybe from Quinn, her black labrador, who was following close behind. That's probably one reason she was pulled in to handle the press. Tom once told her, "You have a strong personality." She believes this may be what contributes to her talent of always being able to complete the task.

She was tapped right away when she started on the Robertson Draw Fire to be in charge of public relations. Lieutenant Hyfield (Amy) had been a first responder and the public information officer in training on the first day of the Robertson Draw Fire. Technically, she was in training the entire "Summer of Hell." She handled public relations for every interview, press release, newspaper article, and social media announcement while also fulfilling her other duties in the field. Amy wears a strong expression proudly, becoming quiet instead of showing tears, holding back as her eyes water with emotion. Her dedication to Red Lodge Fire Rescue is unbounded with time.

As she released the information about Tatum Morrell, she also prepared her SAR team to climb the mountain. The search for Tatum started that day. A crucial lead came when Ivan Kosorok, SAR, saw the page for a missing hiker after returning from his own camping trip nearby. He remembered Tate's tent because she had picked a prime spot and beat everyone to it. It was in a clearing of pine and aspen trees close to a stream, flat, open enough to view the massive granite above that would challenge her hikes, and just enough off the trail for privacy. Ivan also remembered it because no one had come in and out for a few days.

Lieutenant Hyfield led an all-women's hasty team[2] up the mountain to the area described by Ivan. She said it was a good lead, but the crew had less desirable results than expected. They got there before dark. It rained while they were going up, and they were wet. They found her bear bag hanging up, not touched for days. Nine times out of ten, they find the person on the first day. Lieutenant Hyfield thought they would find her. But once they saw her bag, she knew it was bigger than they could handle that evening. They searched the area and yelled, but there was nothing. The four SAR women decided they were cold and wet and needed more personnel. They hiked back out. The National Guard immediately sent in their infrared cameras. They, too, could find nothing.

This second tragedy hit a small town on the edge of wild country—a giant fire burning through town, and now a high-profile missing woman.

The Section House Fire

On July 6, Dan and Katy were still on severity when a third fire, the Section House Fire, took off on the Crow Reservation to the east. Getting there was arduous because of the lack of directions and roads in the vast multi-colored landscape of sandstone, pine, and sage across Crow Country.

Chaos is how every fire must seem to rookie firefighters like Katy, as communications and management expand with every change. Dispatch sends out the initial alert, and fire engines respond. When the command arrives, the right radio frequency is often switched to the color red. Most firefighters have several radios in their vehicles as they monitor several fires simultaneously. Engines from Red Lodge, Joliet, and Bridger responded to this fire on the BLM.

Getting everyone on the same radio channel and setting up the divisions takes time in any fire situation. This one was in the middle of wide, open grass and sage with rough remote canyons and few resources available.

Dan was used to changing communications and management structures as fires expanded. He helped Katy understand that these were potentially the most dangerous moments of firefighting. Roads on the reservation were unknown to non-natives, making it difficult to coordinate any response with other towns. Dan and Katy met with another town's engine and waited for an IC, who would be a Crow native.

"We're gonna start driving up to the fire," said a man from the other engine crew.

"No, you guys need to wait for the Crow IC," said Dan. "We've got an action plan." Crow firefighters are highly respected, but the other engine crew showed impatience. This fire had the potential for a "watch out" situation. Dan couldn't see the fire and waited for the command to scout, size, and plan the attack. His team waited patiently, but the other crew was acting impulsively. Finally, they listened to Dan and waited for the plan. At midnight, heavy equipment arrived to cut a road into the fire so the engines could reach it.

The Pryor Mountains offered a smooth hump outline of the horizon, in shadow of the orange glow of the fire. As Dan and Katy pulled up to the tree line, they realized they could no longer see the stars because they were blocked out by the light of the flames. They couldn't take their vehicles any farther, so they stretched a long line and added another hose length to reach the fire.

As spot fires developed behind them, Katy turned her hose and put them out one after the next. They were cautious because the dark night increased the danger; their instructions were clear, and their escape route was directly behind them.

Katy had the nozzle and started knocking it down. Dan says, "A spot fire broke out behind us; a hand crew was trying to catch it, and it was about to get away from them. Katy spun around and put it out. That was an amazing moment. We were in a tough spot with fires that could have cost us the fire or killed us. On that fire, she became a better firefighter than all the volunteers at our station and many paid people."

Dan stayed on the fire with Katy for four days when Katy left because her mom became sick in Absarokee, Montana. On the fifth day, the fire was almost contained, and Dan returned to the station.

With three fires burning and a missing hiker, Tom, Sarah, Ruth, Jon, and Amy held daily meetings in the firehouse, where they had set up an operations room for the entire summer. Amy says, "The paperwork, the press, the outpouring of support for the fires and Tate never stopped."

In the summer of 2021, Red Lodge had just recovered from the national pandemic. Dan hated the policies that Red Lodge Fire Rescue implemented for COVID-19. EMTs wore masks on calls. Training and learning were remote whenever possible. Most of the Montana State government shut down. Any policy, mask, or vaccine reminded Dan of Marney in the hospital.

Sarah thought the summer was hectic with the fires and the Forest Service in the area to help fight them. An incident management team had been assigned to manage the Robertson Draw Fire while Red Lodge firefighters remained available for other fires and local 911 responses by staying on severity.

On severity with Scott from the 11th to the 15th, Dan was exasperated waiting in the station to be dispatched when fires were already burning. Adding to that was his irritation with the aftermath of a national pandemic.[3]

Sarah describes a no-win situation. "People thought our policy was too much or too lax. We are 911. We have to respond, so we can't get sick. We tried to be strict enough to be safe but loose enough to do our jobs."

Volunteer firefighter Danny Johnson remembers the atmosphere of the firehouse and the town and says that the intensity had grown by July 16. Danny is Tyler's brother-in-law, a fifteen-year member of Red Lodge Fire Rescue. He considers Dan part of the Rae family, as Dan spends most of his time with Tyler and Hank training and fighting fires.

Danny is easily recognizable because his hair gets as messy as his brother-in-law's, and his attractiveness is in his eyes. It is clear he feels everyone's pain. Like all first responders, he would rather have something bad happen to himself than to anyone he loves.

Unaware of his talent for observation and caring temperament, Danny says, "The town was on pins and needles. With the Robertson Draw Fire, because we had lost so much of Mount Maurice, there wasn't much we could do anymore. We worked so hard to be prepared for wildfire, and our ire was up. That fire was as contained as it would be until snowfall."

He adds, "Tom was taking it all hard. He takes things very personally. I could tell he was in rough shape. He was coping, but it was wearing on him. Tate was the rawest for him because she was close in age to his daughters. He takes everything that happens in Red Lodge Fire Rescue personally. The buck stops with Tom."

On July 16, 2021, the big Montana sky was light cyan, and there was an incessant smell of smoke from the east and the south. In the early hours, Red Lodge Fire Rescue was paged to the town of Roberts, thirteen miles north. Dan wasn't on that fire because he was just getting to the station when Tom returned from Roberts.

"Where were you?" Tom asked him, still feeling the weight of the summer.

"I'm on severity today, just getting started," Dan complained as he headed into the firehouse. "How'd it go?"

"A bird hit a power line. It's under control."

"I've been on severity for five days now," Dan said.

"Well, there's lots to do around the station." Tom meant to be reassuring, but his comment seemed to be condescending. Dan refused to look him in the eye and growled under his breath.

"I've been on it long enough. How many weeds can I pull, engines can I shine, or trees can I cut down? It's frustrating," he said. Dan was tired of being on severity, where they spent half the day on fuel crew duty when there were big fires to fight in the rest of the country. He thought it took too much energy from firefighters when they needed to stay rested in case a big fire blew.

Dan looked down at his hands. He was still wearing regular leather gloves to do light mop-ups, equipment checks, and marking timber. To him, this was a waste of his time. He grabbed a cup of water and started to walk away.

"Hey, hold on," said Tom, knowing better than to stop the man by grabbing his arm.

Dan turned around slowly and stood there silently, staring at him, almost daring him to try and say something inspirational. Tom knew

Dan was tough to reach, but he wanted to help if he could. He was pretty good at reading people, and he knew Dan felt underutilized and needed reassurance that he was essential to the team. He thought that Dan struggled to feel purposeful since Marney died. He believed the firefighting organization and its people were even more important to Dan. Tom thought Dan needed to know that the feeling was mutual. He chose his words carefully.

"Hey, the new firefighters look up to you. You are their role model and mentor. I know you want to be out there fighting fires. But we must stay in Red Lodge and Montana to prepare for fires here. We need you here."

Dan didn't answer and returned to the garage. As Tom walked upstairs towards his office, satisfied that he had eased the firefighter's concerns, Dan solely sat on a bench and hung his head. He fought against his truth, which was threatening to reveal itself. He couldn't admit how much he missed Marney, and seeing the COVID masks and vaccines was a constant reminder that she was gone. Fighting big fires would keep those feelings at bay, but working severity was not intense enough to cover up the ache in his heart.

He figured Tom wanted him to feel better and be happy, but that wouldn't happen. He hated being on the sidelines. It was as simple as that, and no amount of brotherly advice or admiration would change anything. Dan stood up and walked around the garage, not feeling any pull to go back in, not feeling any more valued. This "grumpy old man" was on the verge of quitting a job he had worked years to master.

Dan went upstairs to the kitchen, where some of his brothers were cleaning up after breakfast. They all looked up as he entered, and there wasn't a smile in the group.

"Hey, I wasn't done with that," said one of the men to the other.

"Well, hurry up. I'm trying to wash the dishes," said another firefighter.

45

"Whose turn is it to make lunch?"

"You just ate breakfast."

Tim came out of an office and looked around at the surly faces. Knowing severity is painful, he couldn't blame them. Most are grumpy old men who put up with each other, like in any family. No one wants to sit around in a fire station when they should be putting out fires.

Tim saw Dan turn around and head downstairs. "Hey, hold on!" he yelled. Dan stopped, sighed heavily, and waited for him to catch up.

"What's going on, Dan?" Tim asked. "You seem more pissed than usual."

Dan stopped and put his hand up on Engine 78, leaning into it like it was his only friend. "I've been inside long enough. I could be out there teaching Scott and Katy."

Tim opened his mouth to say something motivational, but Dan raised his hand and shook his head to stop him. Without a word, he walked around to the front of the engine to prepare it for its day on severity.

Still off duty, Katy drove to Sheridan, Wyoming, to see a concert with her sister. Captains Rae and Bernard were in Idaho in charge of planning and logistics for the Cougar Rock Complex near Orofino. Amy had traveled to an event out of town.

Sarah listened to the Carbon County Mutual Aid frequency while working at the firehouse. She knew the exact location of her Red Lodge Fire Rescue's engines. Three chiefs (Kuntz, Ryan, Trapp), Ruth, and Danny listened to the same radio frequency.

NWS forecasted potential thunderstorms, which was typical for Montana. Knowing the unpredictable nature of Montana mountains and storms, there was no way to take direct action any more than knowing when to open your umbrella. There was no way to know that today's forecast was monumental.

CHAPTER SIX

"Shit happens fast."

THE NIGHT BEFORE, ON THE 15TH, AROUND MIDNIGHT, A ROGUE lightning strike started a fire on a bluff off of Farewell Road near Joliet, a town about thirty miles north of Red Lodge.

The fire was consuming about three acres in size, a Type 5. The Joliet Fire Department put it out and mopped up for a few hours. As a result, NWS did not know any firefighters were in the area on July 16.

It was midafternoon when Joliet's Chief Melvin Hoferer thought the fire was contained but sent a vehicle back to the site to check for any lingering hot spots. Chief Hoferer (Melvin), in his sixties, standing at 5'7" with graying hair, was a familiar face and had been a fixture of the town of Joliet for decades. His crew reported seeing a curling column of smoke north of town. The fire had reignited. He immediately alerted Carbon County mutual aid radio frequency for help.

Tom's first thought was, "Send Dan. He wants to fight more fires."

When Tim heard the fire dispatched, he agreed. "At least Dan's happy."

Dan and Scott had heard the Carbon County mutual aid radio alert and were already on their way. Engines from Carbon County and Yellowstone County responded, including an engine from the town of Laurel just twelve miles north led by engine boss Captain Sean McCleary. Tall, stout, and solid, Captain McCleary (Sean) was as strong in stature as he was in character and devotion to both his firefighter and blood families. His kindness towards humanity matched his merciless attitude towards wildland fires. When he heard the alert, he knew a fire reigniting just south of his town was trouble.

Sean looked west from his firehouse in Laurel and could just make out a storm gathering west of Park City. He recognized that dry conditions and the potential for incoming strong winds could turn the situation very serious, fast. So he, too, set his sirens, blaring towards Joliet to catch up with all the other engines on the scene, unaware that this horrible season would eventually catch up to him.

The fire was less than a mile west of the Clarks Fork of the Yellowstone River, named after the Lewis and Clark expedition of 1805. It is a tributary of the Yellowstone River system from Yellowstone Park, flowing out of the immense Beartooth Mountains. After Rock Creek meanders and leaves Red Lodge, it joins Clarks Fork of the Yellowstone in a confluence just northeast of Joliet.

At this site, there is an unblemished view of the Beartooth Mountains erupting massively upward from the plains twenty-five miles farther south. From the top of the bluff, the view is of the northern and highest entrance into Yellowstone Park across an ancient glacier glistening in the summer sun. Giant granite spirals seem to hang in the big blue sky above the timberline, snow-packed twelve months a year.

The drama of nature calls the toughest people to settle here and adventurers to witness the grandeur at least once in their lifetime. Ranchers attempt to raise cattle. Antelope roam, eagles soar, and rattlesnakes prosper. Here is where firefighters find unpredictable wind, unburned dangerous sage, grassy fuels of different heights and varieties, and dry humidity early in the season. Even with the Clarks Fork rippling through the yellow grass of the plains, the fire warnings are often bright red, ripe with the potential for catastrophe.

Jeff Brown, a fire management officer with the Department of Natural Resources and Conservation (DNRC) in Billings, was monitoring many radio frequencies when his phone lit up from the IMR—"I am responding"—radio frequency, also known as the Rip and Run, from Carbon County dispatch. Jeff, who Dan thought looked bowlegged, as if he had spent years riding in a rodeo, is six feet tall and slim and conveys a presence of calm authority.

Jeff's first job was to get to a fire site and deal with the first thirty minutes of chaos, mainly getting everyone to switch to the correct color channel: red is command, and yellow is air to ground. Then, he breaks resources into divisions. Jeff had already requested air support to report to command, Chief Hoferer, who directed the helicopter pilot to start dropping water. Driving down Highway 212, Jeff saw the helicopter taking a drop to the other side of the fire.

At 15:38, Dan and Scott were in the first wave of engines on the scene, driving west up Farewell Road just below the bluff, where they could see its edge was on fire with low flames. The chief's plan of attack was to put people underneath and on top of the rim to hold it there. He also called for water drops to dampen the flames and help prevent the fire from progressing down the bluff to Larry Vukonich's farm buildings.

Larry was a very good friend and old neighbor of Dan's. He was in his sixties, a big man, gregarious, smiling, and always ready with a hug for his friends and a story to tell about a lost cow becoming someone's dinner.

At 15:48, the NWS reported the following: "Doppler radar was tracking thunderstorms producing strong wind gusts 11 miles west of

Columbus, moving east at 30 mph. Wind gusts of 50 to 60 mph are possible with these storms. A gust to 63 mph was reported in Big Timber with this activity. Locations impacted include . . . Columbus, Joliet, Absarokee, Reed Point, Halfbreed Lake Wildlife, Park City, Boyd, Molt, and portions of I-90 from Big Timber to Park City."[1]

But this tracking update was not automatically reported to DNRC or Carbon County over the first responder's radios.

Chief Hoferer radioed to the engines below. "Come up to the top of the mesa and put the rest of this fire out."

Dan responded first. He and Scott headed to the top of the bluff.

On top, about four feet wide, one-foot-high flames were going along the edge. From there, Dan could see his friend Larry's old barn in the line of the fire. A couple of miles east was the town of Joliet. He could see the Beartooth Mountains with its white glacier shining above the smoke of the Robertson Draw Fire.

Below the bluff, Larry watched more fire engines racing as fast as they could along the graveled Farewell Road. He did not know his good friend Dan had passed him earlier in Engine 78.

Dan saw an empty big Montana sky as far as he could see to the west. He was aware there had been a thunderstorm warning that morning. But there was none on the horizon. The sky was a uniform bright blue.

Dan and Scott could not see beyond a distant golden bluff that blocked their view of the entire horizon. They didn't see a storm rolling in or know that a deadly wind was building up in front of it—neither did the chief, nor the helicopter pilot in the process of dropping water.

Dan gave the rookie, Scott, specific instructions. "Our escape route is the black. Stay in the truck. Be on the lookout for any change in fire behavior."

Using the hose line from the engine, Dan attacked the grass fire. It had flame lengths of about one to two feet along the bluff edge with a three-hundred-foot plummet down to the fields below. Scott was the lookout, driving the engine as he followed Dan. The fire behavior seemed predictable, with low grass fuel and no wind. Scott could see another small fire miles away to the west. They identified their escape zone as the black from the fire that had been fought the day before. It was a fifty-yard-wide circle directly behind them.

They crossed a barbed wire fence farther into the "green," or unburned fuel. They knew it was risky to go into an open, unburned field, but they stayed in sight of the black, and there was still no wind. They cut a wide swath in the fence so the engine could drive back and forth.

A Joliet engine followed them and headed farther south to attack the mesa's edge from that end. Dan continued to use the hose to push against the low flames as Scott followed in Engine 78.

At 16:14, Jeff was still about five minutes from the site and planned to ask for a spot weather check as soon as he got to the scene. He monitored the weather for seven counties, or what is considered by the DNRC as the Southern Land Office area. He hadn't heard a spot weather report for the area all day. There would be a wind shift sometime in the afternoon, but how significant or from where he didn't know.

As Jeff was about to reach the bluff where the chief, Dan, and Scott were, he was listening to three radios. The helicopter was on one radio frequency, Chief Hoferer on another frequency, and "a bunch" on another.

"I can't see a storm on the horizon, but there is one on radar," said a helicopter pilot. "But it's miles away."

The helicopter was inbound, and the pilots thought the fire was small. "The IC has a plan. We're here. We have some time. We can get some good work done before we bug out." They thought they could help the guys on the ground and were about to tell Chief Hoferer about the storm they could see thirty miles away building on their radar.

Everyone listening on the Carbon County radio frequency was experienced with keeping one ear on the radio and the rest of their attention elsewhere. Sometimes static or a beep and a familiar voice or last name on the radio interrupted them. But mostly, it was noise in the background of their office or vehicle.

At 16:15, they didn't hear what sounded like a freight train crashing on the bluff.

Dan heard it.

It was a wall of a seventy-mile-per-hour wind carrying an erupting volcano.

The downdraft in front of the faraway storm hit hard. The wind came at the helicopter like stampeding buffalo, driving black smoke. The pilot grabbed the switch for an emergency water drop, avoiding slamming into the bluff. The water crashed like a tsunami just south of Dan and Scott's engine. The helicopter blew off the ridge, barely escaping to the grass three hundred feet below.

Dan lost his breath when he saw the helicopter miss their position with the waterfall. He thought of the scene in the movie *Only the Brave* in which the C-130 missed the drop on the Granite Peak Hotshots, which would have dramatically changed their fate. Later, he said, "Funny what you think of when you're running for your life."

He turned and waved his arms vigorously at Scott in the engine. "Head for the black!" he screamed.

Scott slammed his foot on the gas pedal. But it was too late. Flames and smoke swallowed them, blinding and disorienting Scott. He didn't know if he was going towards the black or the bluff's edge. Finally, he hit the brakes and waited for the smoke to clear.

Dan caught up, grabbed the back of the engine, and pressed his body next to the letter E78 just as the monster flames screamed underneath the engine, flashing directly up at him.

Dan put his head down under his helmet and held his breath.

"Oh, shit, this is not going to end well."

He stared into the abyss of yellow, orange, and red for what he thought was an eternity.

His sunglasses protected his eyes.

His simple leather gloves melted away, leaving his hands to blister and peel.

As Dan continued to stare, he felt the inferno consume him as he tried not to inhale death. "Don't breathe, don't breathe," he told himself.

Scott was trapped inside an oven for what he thought was about a minute. The heat inside was like sitting in a roaster pan being basted. Then, as quickly as it had started, it was over, and the smoke cleared. Free from the heat and smoke, he looked out the blackened window and saw Dan, who nodded at him to drive on. He plowed through the fence with his brother firefighter running beside the engine.

Even though he was burned, Dan's mind was only on not getting hurt when he jumped the fence. He kept the hose away from the engine to ensure it did not wrap around the tires and stop them from speeding forward. Then he turned it on the flames that were still burning the engine.

When they stopped in the black, Scott jumped outside the truck and down to the scorched ground, determined to find Dan. "Where are you!" he yelled.

"Scott! I'm over here! Are you all right?" All he was concerned about at that point was Scott's safety. And at first, it seemed like they were both okay.

Dan walked around, shedding his helmet and what was left of his gloves. He took off his melted radio. His boots seemed fine. He looked at his nylon harness, burned beyond black, too hot to touch, and quickly threw it on the fender of the engine.

It was all hot, like grabbing a hot pan from the oven. His radio harness, helmet, and gloves were all burned.

Reluctantly, he said, "Call command and tell them we are out of the fight."

Scott tried twice from the truck radio, but there was no response. So Dan grabbed a hand radio and called Chief Hoferer. "We're burned over! And need help!"

Everyone listening on the Carbon County mutual aid frequency heard the call for help. All over the county, heads bucked up and ears leaned in to hear more clearly as listeners became worried and alert.

At Red Lodge Fire Rescue, Sarah recognized Chief Hoferer's voice on the radio. She didn't know who was hurt or if it was bad. But the Chief sounded more and more frantic. His voice was getting higher pitched. He called for an ambulance, and she assumed it was a Joliet firefighter.

Then she heard Melvin say, "Get your ass here, now."

CHAPTER SEVEN

"Load and Go"

CHIEF HOFERER HAD NEVER BEEN HIT BY A STORM THAT FAST OR hard. He saw the helicopter blast off the bluff, heading straight down. The soot and ashes from the wall of wind hurled him against a tender at the same time. He thought the worst was over. Then he got the call.

"Burned over! Need help."

There was an engine burnover. A firefighter was burned.

He wasn't far from the site. He was there in seconds and saw a burnt, flat pasture still steaming with smoke and water before him. A Red Lodge engine was dead and looked as if it had run aground or charred in a grill, except for the E78 emblem that stood proudly. His heart sank; he dreaded opening the doors and finding firefighters cooked inside.

He saw Scott and Dan standing in the field. His knees buckled. Then, he found a renewed energy and sprang into action. But his elation was short-lived. Scott was okay. But Dan's face was yellow, with pieces melting off. The skin on his back and his legs were blistered and red.

"I felt sick," says Melvin. "First time in thirty-three years that a fireman has been burned on my watch. And it was Dan. It's a small county, and we all know each other. Dan was burned badly. His airway wasn't compromised. I thought they could get him to the hospital. He had protected his airway. He was coherent. He was probably in shock because he didn't realize he was hurt. We all remained calm around him."

Jeff had heard Chief Hoferer asking for help when he was still getting everyone switched to the "Red" radio frequency. Pulling into the black, he saw the IC's truck and the burned engine. Melvin kept his composure, saying calmly that an ambulance was coming.

But Jeff advised against it. "Don't bring the ambulance into the fire, just to the road below." Then he walked over to meet Dan and felt his heart break when he saw his friend. Dan, one of his best students and teacher, with strips of his clothes falling off. His ears, face, and skin were red or ashen and starting to scuff off. His mustache was gone.

Jeff thought at least forty percent of the man before him was burned. They had failed with Order #10. They were not yet fighting fire aggressively and had not had time to provide for safety first.

Dan was alert but lethargic and confused. He kept asking for water. Jeff helped him into his truck and drove him off the bluff to the ambulance waiting below on Farewell Road.

"I fucked up. I fucked up. Water. Water," Dan kept saying on the way down.

At 16:36, Billings Dispatch requested a spot weather check for the Harris Fire. Dan left the scene at 16:50. At 16:55, NWS released an email with their spot weather warning of a strong downdraft near Joliet or the Harris Fire.[1]

Jon first heard a lot of activity on the radio. He, too, heard Melvin request an ambulance. He thought it must have been a landowner who tried to control the fire with a tractor, which often happens. But then he heard the tone of Melvin's voice as it progressed, getting more stressed.

When Jon found out Engine 78 was burned over, his first concern was for Scott because he was brand new, a rookie. So he called him.

"Are you okay?"

"I am," Scott said. "Dan is walking and talking to command, so I think he is okay, too."

The information was spotty at first. Jon thought both men were okay. Then he heard Melvin ask for a rescue flight, which meant it was serious. On top of the Robertson Draw Fire and the search for Tate Morell, the unthinkable had happened. One of their own was burned over on duty.

At that moment, only Melvin and Jeff could see Dan's burns and knew how bad he was. Jeff had called Tim, who had called Tom. The three Red Lodge Fire Rescue chiefs, Tom, Tim, and Jon, remained in the leadership mindset they use to handle crises. Still, they heard the panic and stress in Melvin's voice. And for Dan, "tough" Dan, to agree to get in an ambulance and go to Billings—their emotions were raw. Together, they made a plan. Tom sent Tim to the hospital and Jon to the site.

Joliet Paramedic Marla Frank received the emergency call while at home. Hearing one of their own, a firefighter, was hurt, she called the ambulance station in Joliet and told them to meet her at the scene. St. Vincent's Emergency Room in Billings was almost thirty miles from the fire site by ground, and the weather was not cooperating. Even though Marla and Chief Hoferer had asked for air transport, the same wind and storm that had caused Dan's burns were now determined to delay his journey to get medical attention.

At the scene, Marla looked at Dan's burns, horrific wounds on someone she knew from years on the line together, and gave one command to the team: "Load-n-go."

The twenty minutes it took to make the drive in the ambulance with Dan, going at top speeds with sirens blaring, would change her life. She was afraid he would die before getting to the hospital. Marla had a strong frame of serious determination and a face that could take on the world with its beauty.

Marla wanted to keep him talking to listen for any change in his voice, any sign that his airway had collapsed.

"Dan, tell me about your family. Who should we contact?" Marla asked over the siren's noise.

"Call my sister. This will be too upsetting for my daughter. Here, let me give you my password for my phone. Where is my phone?"

It wasn't the smoothest ride. Highway 212 has a few bumps before it gets to I-90, and even that has rough, weathered dips. They would both bounce up as they tried to communicate.

Marla wanted to cut off the rest of his shirt and pants. Dan said, "I can take them off." During the jostling ride, he adjusted his body to remove his clothes.

"Let me get your boots."

"They cost $600. Fuck no. My feet aren't burned," Dan said.

Taking off his boots, Dan said, "Honestly, it's not that bad. I can probably go home."

Marla tried to help him with his boots, but he shooed her hands away. "I can do it!"

She could only stay calm and keep him talking.

Dan was alert and had no idea he was severely hurt. His main concern was for his firefighter brothers. "Make sure they know I'm okay. Take care of themselves on the fire."

As she kept him talking, she alerted St. Vincent's Hospital of his status to prepare them for the severity of his burns. Marla could see blisters all over Dan's body, and his face was extremely white.

She finally found a vein in his arm through his burned skin, to give him fluid from an IV. If he stopped breathing, Marla was ready to intubate him; if that didn't work, Marla had a trach ready. She kept her voice calm on the radio to the ER at St. Vincent's so that Dan did not feel her stress.

She tried to prepare him for what was ahead at the hospital. "You will be intubated. You will be going to a burn center. You are badly burned," Marla told him steadily. The trip with Dan was one of two times in her career that she was in the ambulance with someone she thought would die.

Dr. Kathi Theade was waiting at St. Vincent's Emergency Room, listening to Marla's voice on the radio. The doctor's appearance is deceptive with her perfect button nose, high cheekbones, and slight frame. Her sweet, friendly voice hid the mighty package of the life-saving emergency doctor and leader who didn't blink. "First responders are part of our very small circle," she says about Marla. "It is very difficult to put our personal feelings on the shelf. As soon as my paramedic is nervous, I know the patient coming in is very sick."

They knew each other very well, and Dr. Theade could hear the quivering in Marla's voice. "The more critical the situation, the more clipped and pressured the voice tone. I can feel her putting away any personal emotional response to focus on the problem. We call this the game face. I got this from Marla as she brought Dan to me. The stress in her voice but complete attention to the task despite knowing him personally."

Dr. Theade agreed with Marla's initial assessment. "When I first saw him, I thought this was as bad as Marla said. My eyeballed, quick calculation of the percentage was at least sixty percent of his body. Strips of skin were falling away. His mustache was gone, and his lips and ears were badly burned. Now, I'm thinking through the differential diagnosis and preparing mentally. In Dan's case, it's easy to see the obvious injury, the burns. Could he have suffered a medical emergency like a heart attack that prevented him from escaping the flames? I found out later that he was on rheumatoid arthritis medication, making him very susceptible to infection. My job as a leader is quickly assessing this and knowing what intervention I will perform. The nurses quietly laid out their IV setups, the bladder catheter, the dressings, the pharmacist gathered the drugs we'll need, the respiratory therapist prepared the equipment they already know I'll need to intubate and double checking it all. Radiology techs already have the X-ray plates in the slots under the gurney, my techs ready to transfer Dan, place him on monitoring and, because we are St. Vincent's, our chaplain was in attendance to not only give comfort but to receive and coordinate care for Dan's family and the EMS crew affected."

The swarm of medical personnel is what Dan saw as he was rolled in from the ambulance, strapped to a gurney. So many strangers in their scrubs and masks were waiting for him. He wanted to scream at them that he wasn't hurt. Dan hates a fuss. He hated hospitals. But seeing everyone's seriousness in this emergency room, he thought maybe he was hurt and wondered how badly.

Behind the masks and scrubs of the doctors and nurses in the room, he could see eyes that expressed more than concern. He saw fear, as if they were watching someone die. Could he be dying?

"Don't leave me alone," he told Marla as she left.

"Only family can stay now," she said, grabbing his hand.

"You *are* my family."

Marla steadied her breathing. Tears built up in her eyes and rolled down her cheeks. But she stayed calm for Dan.

Dr. Theade's team took their collective breath before unstrapping Dan from the gurney. "Everyone, with quiet words of encouragement and reassurance to Dan, did what we do best. There's a quote from a book written in the 70s by Samuel Shem called *The House of God*. I think of it every time. 'The first pulse you take in a code is your own.'"

The ballet of saviors began restoring life to every critical need before them. "The tricky fact about critical burns is that they are not painful because the skin that has sensation is burned away. The patient often talks calmly, unaware that their skin hangs off their body in strips and their ears are missing parts," says Dr. Theade. "Without the protective barrier of the skin, fluid losses are enormous. However, the single most important intervention that will save a life in a critical burn is securing the airway by intubating [putting a breathing tube in through the mouth into the lungs] quickly. Why? If I see soot in the back of the throat or burns inside the mouth, I can be sure the breathing airways have been burned, and in a very short time, they will swell suddenly, cut off breathing, and my patient will die."

When Tim reached the ER, he looked around in bewilderment at the surrounding blue-scrub-clad strangers, probing his friend.

"I'm sorry, I fucked up. I'm sorry, I fucked up," said Dan, reaching out for him.

Tim leaned in beside his brother and saw what everyone saw. Dan's skin was peeling from his arms, legs, and ears. His hair and mustache were gone. Tim held back a gasp and tried to reassure him. "Don't worry about it. We're just going to take care of you."

"Can you find my wallet? It's in my pants pocket," Dan said.

Dan's clothes had been carefully cut away; Tim found them in the biohazard bag underneath the gurney. The back of his pants was so badly burned that there were no pockets. There was no wallet. "Dan, I'm afraid your pockets are gone, but I'll find your wallet."

Tim was just trying to hold it together, not to upset Dan. He had been dealing with this "shit" all his life because, like many firefighters, he had a medical background. The hospital team told Tim they estimated Dan had third-degree burns on over sixty percent of his body, and he was scheduled for the next flight to Utah.[2]

Dr. Theade was "the captain of the ship," remaining calm because everyone fed off her emotions. Overly calm. She got about six inches from Dan's face and explained, "I am going to sedate and intubate you. I promise I will keep you comfortable no matter what. You will wake up again in the Salt Lake City burn unit. Don't be afraid. We all will do our best. You can trust us."

Dan remembers she was direct and used few words. "I liked that."

Dr. Theade remembers Dan looking straight into her eyes and saying, "If you knew what I've been through in my life, you'd know I'm not afraid to die."

Dan's words startled the doctor. "I almost lost it when he said that to me. I was proud of Dan, that he was so cooperative, engaging with people. His courage was profound. *He* was reassuring *me*. He was so calm and accepted every step and that his fate was in someone else's hands." Dr. Theade also thought his lack of fear saved him because adrenaline can work against someone who has been burned so badly. "Being able to face forward calms you. It had a lot to do with his recovery."

The courage behind his statement affects Dr. Theade to this day. She thought he was referring to surviving heartache and overcoming tragedies. Dan said, "I'm still not afraid to die because I've lived through and done everything I can imagine doing."

Dan scanned the room, making eye contact with everyone. Now, there were tears along with the fear he had seen. *Were these his last words?* He said, "Thank you, each and every one of you."

Then, for Dan, the room went black.[3]

CHAPTER EIGHT

Heavy Hearts

Dan was intubated, IV lines were connected, and fluids were checked, following a well-established protocol for air transport. The energy was fast-paced but meticulous as the medical team readied Dan for the flight to Salt Lake.

Then it seemed like suddenly the world had stopped. There was an empty place in the middle of the room where Dan's gurney had been, with the tubes and cords unhooked and dangling.

A steel table held a messy collection of instruments, tin containers, discarded gowns, and a box of blue latex gloves. The polished reflection of the floor was sullied with dropped bandages, used tissues, and disposable masks.

Everyone stood around, almost shocked by the changing atmosphere that had quickly turned from a well-rehearsed medical symphony with every instrument in perfect tune to dead silence. Marla stared blankly at the mess. The EMTs that broke records to get Dan to Billings stood frozen, heads down and arms wound across their chests, hugging their hearts. Dr. Theade took a deep breath, feeling her adrenaline dwindle. She knew everyone on her staff felt the same release, but it was time to clean up, so she gave the orders.

Marla snapped out of her haze and looked around, panic setting in her eyes as she tried to squelch the hysteria rising up through her body. Suddenly, she couldn't keep it in any longer and bolted out of the room into the hallway. From the bottom of her stomach, she felt the anguish coming up and then out of her head. She lost control and bawled loudly.

Tim followed her and found the entire ambulance crew was visibly shaken. No one was immune to their nerves exploding after staying calm in order to do their critical care job. Dr. Theade came out of the room and put her hands squarely on Marla's shoulders, trying to comfort her. "You did everything right. You kept him alive and got him here."

Marla had been caring for one of her own, another first responder. Every ounce of her strength had been focused on her training, staying calm, keeping her voice steady, prepping the hospital, keeping Dan talking, and finding the one spot in his destroyed skin for an IV. She had watched over him blistered and melting away, ready with a tube or trach at hand.

Tim tried to console Marla but could no longer hold it himself. A member of their family was very likely dying. Dan may have just spoken his final words to Tim. And, of course, as it was Dan, it was full of cursing. Tim wished he had offered something more. So much was left unsaid about family, love, respect, and honor.

Firefighting then became very real to Tim. He thought about how lucky everyone had been. So many times, it could have happened to any of them; it was all fortune, or lack thereof. His mind became inundated with the many close calls throughout the years. The images of wind and flames came to him vividly, over and over. It could have been a rookie. It could have been someone he trained. These thoughts would never leave Tim's head. And he cried. He thought of Dan's hands and how burned they were. And he kept crying.

It would be another year before Marla got back into an ambulance. The stress of keeping it together, of keeping Dan alive long enough to get him to Dr. Theade, had been one of the hardest moments of her life. If Dan had died, she later said, "I would have given up the job."

Back on Farewell Road, Jeff had moved on to a second fire near Huntley, the Buffalo Fire. He couldn't stop for emotions as he was dealing with the facts of an injured man and two new fires. Chief Hoferer also had to keep his feelings in check, as he was still fighting the Harris Fire.

"I had to snap out of it and keep being an IC. The size and intensity of the Harris Fire took my attention away until a couple of days later. Structures were in danger, and there was an out-of-control fire headed for the town. We evacuated Joliet. I couldn't dwell on Dan for the first couple of days."

Jon arrived on the scene. He was relieved to see Scott healthy, using a hand tool on the edge of the black, putting out any leftover flames. Scott had been waiting an hour beside burned-over Engine 78. Both he and Jon were concerned for Dan, knowing it had to be bad if Dan agreed to leave in an ambulance. Jon took a moment to examine the inside of the fried engine and found Dan's phone still on the seat.

With his own phone, Jon took a photo of the dead E78 and sent it to Tom.

Tim gathered his thoughts enough to call Tom. He described the scene in the ER and told him that Dan was in critical condition and didn't know if he would even make it to Utah. He could sense Tom, who had received the photo from Jon, putting his head in his hands on the other end of the line, knowing both of them were now letting tears silently run.

Tom hung up the phone and wiped his tears. He kept looking at the photo of E78 on his phone. He leaned his head way back until his mouth gaped open, wanting to scream, but instead taking noisy breaths. He threw his head forward and looked again at the photo. He forcefully pushed his chair back from the desk until his arms were straight. Then, with one movement, he stood strong, gathering his courage, knowing he had to tell Sarah. He also knew it would be especially rough.

She stood at the open door to his office; her face was in shadow, but he knew she was waiting for him to speak. All he needed to say was, "It's Dan."

Her heart dropped into her stomach. Her knees buckled. It could not be Dan. *He cannot be dying tonight. There was still so much left unsaid between us. Did he know how much I loved him as my dearest friend and member of my family? Did I put my arms around him enough to show him he was safe at Red Lodge Fire Rescue? It just cannot be Dan.*

She calmed herself and put on a stoic front. She knew there was work to do to support Dan and all the Red Lodge Fire Rescue firefighters. Instead of falling apart, she got to work.

On his way back to the firehouse, Tim stopped at the scene, needing to salute or pray to the burned and destroyed E78. As he walked in a circle around this oven with wheels, crunching the black grass beneath his boots, he found Dan's wallet on the ground about fifteen feet away, completely intact.

Tim, Jon, Tom, and Sarah started making all the tough calls and announcements. Jon called Cindy Northey, Dan's older sister.

"I've got some severe news about Dan. He's been in a burnover. He's all right, but he's on a life flight to the burn center in Utah."

Cindy wanted to be strong for Dan. She felt a tremendous responsibility to notify the rest of the family for him. Later, she would say,

"That he would give me that responsibility was an honor. I would make sure I did it the way he wanted me to. I stayed strong."

Her first call was to Susie Steffensen, the mother of Hannah and Will. She delivered the news to Hannah, who immediately called Will. All three made arrangements to fly to Salt Lake City the next day.

Most firefighters would not officially know what had happened for another hour because the names of burn victims are never said on the radio. Most engine crews in the county knew that Roberts and Red Lodge engines had joined the firefight in Joliet. They heard about Engine 78, which meant Red Lodge; that day, it was Dan and Scott.

Much of Tom's emotional distress was because he knew burn victims are considered "the walking dead." They seem fine at first because they cannot feel pain. Then, they deteriorate until they are dead. Just that morning, Tom told Dan how important he was to the Red Lodge Fire Rescue. At 7:51 p.m., he sent out an email.

From: messaging@iamresponding.com
Date: July 16, 2021, at 7:51:32 PM MDT
Subject: FD7-Red Lodge
It is with a heavy heart that I need to inform everyone that E78 with Scott Wilson and Dan Steffensen was burned over earlier today on the Harris Fire in Joliet. Fortunately, Scott was not injured. However, Dan Steffensen suffered severe burn injuries and was transported to Billings and later flown to Salt Lake City. We will keep in touch as more information becomes available. Please keep Dan in your thoughts and prayers -Tom.

News spread everywhere, fast. Captain Bernard received a message on his cell phone while at the Cougar Complex ICP in Orofino, Idaho, that there had been a burnover involving Red Lodge Fire Rescue personnel. He called Tim, who told him it was Dan. Will's heart stopped beating. Dan was his student who always tried to do everything perfectly—so much so that Dan now trained and mentored the new recruits. *What went wrong? Did I not teach him enough?*

Jon's photo of burned Engine 78 had reached Salt Lake Unified Fire Authority (UFA) Wildland Division Chief Anthony Widdison, making UFA Chief Dan Petersen aware of an on-duty burnover in Montana. Chief Petersen knew Chief Kuntz at Red Lodge from their Western Fire Chiefs Association work.

"I consider Tom a friend," said Chief Petersen. "He is called on often because he can see clearly and wants to be part of the solution. He's a good partner." Even though he was from a small organization, Chief Kuntz was well respected and involved in national wildland issues and on important committees nationwide.

Chief Petersen had experienced and felt the grief himself and wanted to help. "When I heard he had a man coming to Utah, I reached out. I could sense he was shaken, and I just wanted to take something off his plate and let him know about my resources here."

Will's next call was to Tom, who told him that the UFA Honor Guard would receive Dan and implement their Honor Guard protocol. Tom said, "One of us has to be there. Dan is our man. Our family." Will agreed.

Tom couldn't get to Salt Lake City until 4:30 the following afternoon. Will found a flight leaving Lewiston, Idaho, that would get him to Salt Lake City at 8:30 a.m. Tom contacted UFA, arranged transportation for Will from the airport to the hospital, and planned to meet him the next day.

Will spoke with his Idaho IC and explained the situation and the plan. Idaho had one response: "We will make it happen." Dan's friend, Captain Rae, was managing logistics on the same fire. As much as he wanted to be with Dan, he and Will could not be released simultaneously. They decided they would tag-team. When Will returned to Idaho, Tyler would go to Utah.

Tom's email went out, but Katy didn't see it because she was having dinner with her sister in Sheridan, Wyoming. Instead, she got a text from a search and rescue crew member, Dani Cunningham.

Are you OK?

Yeah, Fine.

I just heard from a law enforcement friend that a Red Lodge engine was burned over. I heard Dan was hurt. I thought you were with Dan. I heard they took him to the hospital.

Katy immediately excused herself from the table, went outside, and texted Red Lodge Fire Rescue firefighter Jozee Plouffe, who was fighting the Robertson Draw Fire. When she confirmed that Dan was hurt, Katy called her.

"He was burned over. It was Dan and Scott. They couldn't use air support to Billings, but they are flying him to Utah," Jozee told her.

Katy slid down to the sidewalk, clutching the phone against her ear. Gathering her power, she returned to the table. She tried to be calm, but her sister could tell something was wrong.

"It's Dan," Katy told her. "I don't know how bad it is. I can't eat."

She texted Jon's wife for news, and he called her back. "He's intubated, and they are flying him to Salt Lake."

Katy knew that meant Dan was in terrible shape. She had to get back home. She had to get air. There was a lone corner on the street where no one could see her. She ran to it as her sister took care of the check and raced for the car.

It was on a street corner in Sheridan. Katy let it go.

Her concern for Dan turned to guilt. *I should never have taken a day off. I should have been there. He's my best friend. My mentor. Not Dan.* She felt as though mud were rising from her stomach to her throat, so thick she couldn't move her jaw to gag. Her mouth was wide open with no sound, and tears fell down her cheeks.

Then she stopped, knowing Dan would not want this. She wiped them off with the palm of her hand, one cheek at a time. She allowed one large sniff.

As Dan's plane left Billings airport, her sister drove her back to Greybull, Wyoming, where she picked up her truck. She turned on the engine and placed her forehead between her hands on the top of the steering wheel. If she had let go again, the neighbors would have thought they heard a coyote howling from her mournful crying. Instead, she drove back to Red Lodge, gathered her EMS and wildland gear, and drove to the station.

Katy said, "I had a job to do. I knew I had to be strong for everyone." That is what Dan would have wanted.

CHAPTER NINE

"Well fuck"

CAPTAIN ANTHONY WIDDISON RACED ALONG I-15 TO THE UNIVER-
sity of Utah Health Burn Center (UUBC) from his home, an hour away.
It wasn't the first and wouldn't be the last time he rushed to assist Utah's
Unified Fire Authority (UFA), an organization involved in everything
from first response and transport to dealing with bomb threats. In
one year alone, the UFA answered 35,972 emergency incidents and
assisted twenty-four fire stations with 64,294 unit responses. He'd seen
lives go from safe to destroyed in an instant. He'd seen trauma explode
into tragedy. And he'd seen pain.

But this one felt personal.

Captain Widdison (Anthony or Wood) knew he was needed when
he saw the photo of the blackened E78 from Red Lodge. He wanted to
be there for his firefighter brother. "I thought a firefighter was coming
from that vehicle, burned on duty. He will be away from family. I had
to help receive him."

Several others were getting ready for Dan's arrival in Salt Lake City.
Assistant Chief Riley Pilgrim was also on the way to the burn center
to help make sure all resources were in place. Captain Jared Wayman,
UFA Honor Guard, and firefighter, got Anthony's call for the Honor

Guard to be on standby, and Captain Tommy Miller joined him. Captain Wayman's dedication to making the Honor Guard as essential to the job as a tender or an engine was unmistakable. His time belonged to every firefighter and their family. His heart was open with arms stretched wide enough to hold a thousand survivors.

Dan arrived in Salt Lake City around 2:00 a.m. on July 17. After several cups of coffee, the UFA firefighters anxiously waited in the ambulance bay. The ambulance doors ground loudly open as Dan was pulled out on his gurney. Captain Wayman (Jared) and Captain Miller (Tommy), in full-dress uniform, were there to stand with him.

Anthony helped pull the gurney from the ambulance. Anthony's manner was deceptively peaceful. Underneath his calm smile was a man respected for leadership, intelligent planning, and strength in a wildland firefight. He proudly wore a bald head atop his strong physique. But the sight of the burned firefighter shook his strong exterior. When the three seasoned firefighters first saw Dan and the extent of his injuries, they were sure they were looking at a dying brother. "It was an impossibility. We just looked at each other and then bowed our heads," says Anthony.

Captain Wayman agreed. "We were pretty sure the man we saw being rushed to his room would die soon. We were not going to leave his side."

Anthony has a flight paramedic background and observed Dan as he came off the ambulance intubated with pumps attached for breathing. "I could see that his burns were more developed than most. He was on the transport ventilator, and his IV pumps provided the medication for sedation and pain. I saw his face. The skin was flaking off. It was bright pink with ashen areas. His face and lips were swollen."[1]

Anthony helped with the gurney all the way to the ICU room and helped lift Dan to the bed. "I was concerned. A facial burn usually means internal bronchial burns. Everyone in medical was super focused, debriding, washing with the rags, and cleaning it all off. Jared and Tommy were the Honor Guards. I was just there as a representative for Dan and Riley."

Captains Wayman and Miller were in ceremonial dress uniform, double-breasted with gold buttons, with shined shoes and white covers with gold trim, lovely, tragic, as they stood, never faltering, outside the heavy wooden double doors of Dan's ICU room. Through the tall glass windows of the doors, they were witness to their dying brother at first on his back, then rolled to one side and then the next, as the torture team of doctors scrubbed the burned skin from his body.

The first nurses ensured all IVs were in place, cleaned as much of the burns as possible, and did a complete wrap-up. "They let the burns sit, letting the burn declare if the skin will be dead or alive," explains Nurse Erik Mandeen.

Burns are terrible and traumatic for the skin and everything beneath. Second degree is the most painful. Third—the nerves are gone. The medical team cleans the burned and dead top layer of skin off to limit infection before they wrap him like a mummy. The question is whether the lower layers will live or not. Surgery will then remove dead tissue.

Erik had heard the call about Dan coming. "When they told me a firefighter was arriving, a patient aged sixty-five, with sixty percent burn size, on rheumatoid arthritis medicine Methotrexate, which compromised his immune system, I knew I had to take the call. His odds of surviving the first day or two were low." Erik was determined Dan would live while on his watch. "We knew he was going to be a very sick patient."

Assistant Chief Pilgrim (Riley) met Will at the Salt Lake City airport and drove him to see Dan in the burn center. Riley wore a face that showed he cared about people to a fault. "My heart breaks when I see a tragedy like this occur with another firefighter. I wanted to ensure Dan and his family's life was as good as possible. That is all that matters."

Riley told Will his friend was in bad shape, and he tried to prepare him for the shock. It was the first time Will stood outside and covered himself in paper gowns, booties, masks, and caps. It wouldn't be the last. When Will entered the room, he stopped breathing, seeing Dan, a tall, tough guy, wrapped, intubated, and not responding. "There were two slits in the bandages around his head for his eyes. His arms, legs, and hands were also bandaged. I wasn't sure he could hear my voice. But I kept it together. I didn't want him to think, from my reaction, that it was as bad as I knew it was. At that point, I wasn't sure he would last until Tom arrived later that afternoon."

There was one armchair in the corner and more wooden folding chairs with white upholstery in the closet across from the bed. Will unfolded a chair and pulled it up beside Dan's bed. He talked to Dan, told some jokes, and touched him on the only place he could find that wasn't burned to let him know he was there.

Erik, a firefighter, was a big guy with a matching smile. He assured Will that Dan could hear him. And Will thought his friend responded because his eyes would look in his direction when he spoke. He also believed he saw traces of a smile from Dan in response to some of his "off-color" humor, the kind he knew Dan would appreciate.

As his first full-day nurse, Erik was pissed when a team of ophthalmologists came to check on the patient, and a resident walked in and pried Dan's eyes open.

"Well, does he show any discomfort in the eyes?" he asked Erik.

"He's awake, so ask him." The resident jumped back, as he had assumed Dan was sedated, then was reprimanded by the senior attending for prying a patient's eyes open without all the information. Erik then told the resident to always assume the patient was awake.

Dan's eyes were swollen from the burns and in some pain, but they were in good shape because of the sunglasses he had been wearing during the burn. And his face was not so burned that it had to be grafted.

Dan struggled all day because of the pain and discomfort of raw burns covered with gauze. When Tom arrived, he thought Dan might not make it through the night. The medical staff met with all of them in the hallway outside Dan's room. They told Will and Tom that Dan was far from out of the woods.

When they left later that night, both looked back through the glass on the doors. Tom touched the glass, and Will put his hand on Tom's shoulder. They might have been praying because they were silent in their belief that it could be the last time they'd see him.

The Honor Guard was posted with Dan all night as he slept. Tommy, a strong man at 6'4" and 280 pounds, was one of the people there to protect their brother. "They let us into the room individually. A student nurse was trying to staple something to his head. She kept missing, and I saw Dan wince every time." Finally, Tommy told her to stop. "We're done. You're out. You're not practicing on my brother."

Tommy stood guard in the room as Riley took Will and Tom to dinner in the hospital cafeteria. Riley offered to explain everything that would happen and how Red Lodge Fire Rescue needed to prepare.

"Dan had nothing to do with their department, but Riley took him and us into their family that night," says Will. "He told us what to expect for how to handle our department. He gave us a road map for what we had never experienced and talked about the support we needed to give Dan, including how to care for his house, family, and finances. Dan would leave the life he had for a long time, and we would take care of it. But also, our department would be affected, and we needed to take care of ourselves."

Before that night, Red Lodge Fire Rescue leadership did not have the experience of dealing with a situation like Dan's. "I believe the genesis of everything Red Lodge Fire Rescue subsequently did as a department to support Dan, his family, and the members of Red Lodge Fire Rescue, as well as communicate with our community, was the conversation that Riley and Tom had that night," says Will.

The conversation occurred over a two-hour dinner, sharing cafeteria food and experiences from similar situations involving the 700-member UFA department. Will says, "Tom listened, asked the right questions, and appreciated the guidance. Everything started that night. I don't think I will ever forget those couple of hours."

In ICU, Utah's Dr. Giavonni Lewis wore matching turquoise glasses, scrubs against her dark skin, and her always brilliant smile. But her face was serious when she realized that Dan could be a member of "the walking dead." She planned to remove the burn tissue immediately to reduce stress from the burn on his internal organs. Dan's burn diagram showed which shaded areas were full thickness, which meant they would require surgery to cut away the burn tissue and, eventually, skin grafts to close the burn wounds. She prepared Dan for surgery that night.

"We want excision and allografting within two days of the injury, which starts at the time of the incident," says Dr. Lewis. "We accomplished that for Dan's posterior neck, back, and buttocks. Within five days, we had done his abdomen and anterior legs. Dan was excised entirely within the first five days."

When Will gowned up and walked in the next day, he was pleasantly surprised by Dan's "holy cow" improvement. He had more range of motion, attentiveness, and responsiveness than the previous day. Will grabbed Tom's arm, and Tom grabbed back as they watched Dan move, trying to communicate.

They told him everyone was asking about him, and the texts and calls hadn't stopped. Will asked Dan if there was anything he wanted to say to everyone back home. Dan waved his hand for a magic marker and whiteboard, then slowly but very legibly wrote two words.

"Well fuck."

Their spirits were high from the famous words that Dan had uttered in training and on incidents when he had not performed to his perfect expectations.

"I knew that under all that gauze was Dan. He was still there," says Will. "I laughed. I felt so much better."

Dan signaled he wanted to know how long he would be in Utah. Erik looked at each firefighter in the room and put his hands together as if to pray, silently indicating that their brother would need emotional support. He then told the patient it would be some time. Dan fell back, deflated. He dropped his head into the same lack of responsiveness as the day before.

Tom and Will worried he was giving up. Erik said, "Dan, look at me. Do you think you're the first person that's been here? You and I have a job to do. We are going to start working. A lot of that time is physical therapy. It's up to you. We've got work to do, and I will be with you for the entire time."

Erik explained later how excruciatingly slow this process can be. "A 60% burn is estimated to be in the hospital for four to six months. But you can't tell them that. You have to tell them to focus on this week and next week. How long is what every burn patient wants to know. It destroys them. Their will goes away at that point. Dan was a salty dog. So, I talked to him as a firefighter. I told him this is like a big brush fire you can't think of months later. You need to think of it as operational periods. What's the goal for today, this week, and next week? No further. And he seemed to think he could do that. Getting through this day was all I was thinking because I knew Dan was fucked up."

Dan lifted his head and put his hand out towards Erik. Erik lightly touched him back on top of the bandage. There was a visible rise in Dan's slanted posture. He was okay for the moment.

Erik took everyone into the hall for a truth session. "We won't know for a few weeks if he is out of the woods. It's up to Dan. Our job is to keep him up. But it's up to him to keep going."

When they returned to the room, Dan wrote Will a note asking about Scott and was relieved to find out he was fine. Then he wrote, "Time for you to go." Will knew what it meant. Dan was telling him, "I've got work to do, and so do you. You came. Thanks. I'll see you later." Even when he couldn't talk, his few written words were meaningful.

Support for Dan was coming in from everyone. Erik received a phone call from his old firefighter boss in New Jersey, who was actively deployed on a fire. "Please tell Dan's family that the Jersey crew is rooting for him."

News of Dan's plight had already crossed the country. "Dan's case touched everyone because it is a big deal when a wildland firefighter gets burned over. They normally don't survive, let alone make it to a burn center as bad as he was," Erik says.

While Tom and Will were in Utah, the mood at Red Lodge Fire Rescue was somber and quiet. On her first day back, Katy walked into the station's garage, knowing Dan wasn't there but still searching for him, as if he might be prepping E78.

It was gone, too.

She held back a tear when she saw Assistant Chief Jim Avent. Katy tried to keep her composure as she realized he wasn't smiling like usual. Two upbeat and happy people were shaken that morning. They both choked up. In silence, Jim leaned on one of the bay pillars, and Katy leaned against the bumper of A71.

In the firehouse, Danny held his coffee cup with both hands, twisting it around without picking it up to take a drink. "I felt so bad when I found out it was Dan. My family, Tyler and Hank, spent the most time training Dan. I knew this was going to hit them hard."

Danny had talked to Tyler on the phone. He tried to comfort Tyler, who was in rough shape. "We both cried when we found out it was Dan. We know it's possible. But not Dan. Please, not Dan. I would rather it had been me."

Will returned to his fire assignment in Idaho, and Tyler headed to Utah with every doubt and regret running through his mind. His friend and mentee was, by then, in a coma. "I thought I hadn't taught him enough. It was my fault. I just wanted to sit next to him," said Tyler. "Any moment he would wake up, we would talk about how to fight fires again. The man I was sitting next to could not be my friend. He was helpless. He was unrecognizable. I felt guilty."

Tom returned to Red Lodge and called everyone into the firehouse to tell them that Dan was stable and in good spirits but had a long road ahead. When he shared Dan's "Well fuck" photo, it was the first time everyone had hope. From that moment, Red Lodge Fire Rescue and the community went to work to implement everything Tom had learned from his colleagues at the UFA.

In Utah, Dan's "blood" family had already arrived as separately as they lived. His daughter Hannah and son Will were close as brother and sister. Marney's daughters, Mandy and Margot, were sisters and each other's best friends. Dan's brother, Kelly Steffensen, had not been close to any of them for years. Overall, they were not close to each other or even to Dan. They lived far enough, long enough away that they had no experience with the sacrificial life of a firefighter's family.

The Honor Guard would meet them at the airport, lend them their cars, and hold their hands when they worried about Dan's future. Layne counseled them as they shared their regrets and hopes. With their physical and emotional distance from Dan and each other, they came into Utah utterly blind to what was about to happen to them.

These good, caring, and intelligent individuals would now face their first experience as a firefighter family together. The worst trauma possible gave them no choice but to hold on to each other fast.

CHAPTER TEN

All in the Family

DAN WAS NEVER LEFT ALONE.

Dan's eyes would be shut for weeks; he couldn't see how far his family had all come for him. They were almost strangers when they walked onto the ICU floor. But now, they all had one purpose: to save the man lying in the hospital bed.

The Honor Guard had tried to prepare them to see Dan completely wrapped, with an endotracheal tube down his throat. Dan's daughter Hannah, sharing the same big smile and strong forehead as her mother, didn't want to leave him. But the rest of the family was waiting for her. She lightly touched her lips to his forehead. He was completely out.

"Everyone's out there, Dad. I've got to go talk to them," she said.

Hannah opened the heavy wooden doors of his room and turned the corner of the hall out the security door to the tiny waiting room area. She panned the room. The Honor Guard stood as she approached them. She grabbed Jared's hand and held it for a moment. Her brother got a cup of coffee from the family kitchen area, stirred in cream, and handed it to their mother. Her uncle Kelly was talking to one of the doctors.

"I'll go in now," Will said.

Hannah reassured him. "I think he knows we are here. Just touch his hand and talk to him."

Hannah was surprised to see Mandy and Margot. She smiled at them. The two sisters seemed to magically move in sync toward Hannah and meet in the middle of the room. She leaned into them, and the three women embraced each other in a wide circle without words.

Mandy was a 5'4" brunette who constantly exercised and stayed busy raising a teenage son. Margot was a pensive 5'7" blonde with a teenage daughter. While Mandy described herself as filling space with noise, Margot was quiet. When she talked, people listened. The two sisters were different people and still best friends.

Margot and Mandy were told about Dan and didn't hesitate. "This was a big fucking deal. We got a plane immediately," says Mandy. "Margot and I gave Hannah some space for a day."

The sisters arrived through the Burn Center's security and construction maze. It was not how they planned to reunite with the family. "We weren't not going to be there," says Mandy. "There had been a distance between us, but we loved him. He had cared for our mother; we owed him."

When Dan's sister Cindy told them that Dan had been burned over, Hannah and her mother were "shocked." They didn't realize he was that close to the flames. He had told them he had become a firefighter but let them believe he just drove the tenders.

Hannah, who had Dan's power of attorney, was a young woman with young children and a responsible job at Kroger that she left behind to be with her father. Her internal strength was evident with every step, walking into a meeting or hiking on a trail. She would draw on it now as never before.

"All of sudden, Hannah was dealing with everyone: her mother, all the family, firefighters, medical, logistics, and financials," says Mandy. "She was constantly inundated. She was amazing. She stepped up and took charge of everything for Dan."

Margot says, "When I saw him, I thought, 'I'm not sure this is better than dying.'"

Layne helped them hold vigil in the ICU. He says they were distinct individuals, all loving, intelligent, and determined people. Each one had their own story of their relationship with Dan, and regrets came to the surface for all of them. There was more to tell him, more to show him. Time, communication, and distance had created a chasm in their connections.

Layne, who was also burned on his face, remembers how hard it was for his family to get the news he was hurt. But he was able to go home that same night. Everyone close to Dan was going to be traumatized for months. Most firefighter families are torn apart with worry, and it's easy to question why anyone would do this. Is it worth it? Layne and the Honor Guard helped Dan's family try and understand the choice of being a firefighter.

"Even the horrible things I've seen or injuries I've sustained. I wouldn't change a thing. I'm comfortable with my training," says Layne. "To be in danger and come out unharmed even when it doesn't always go as planned—the reward is knowing you made a difference and helped someone, knowing that you were there for someone on their worst day."

As an Honor Guard, Riley understands the burn community more than most. "The most shitty moments of someone's life, I can make it less shitty. It frustrates my family sometimes that I do a better job or am more empathetic to strangers. I will move heaven and earth for them. But I want my kids to learn to solve their own problems. A bad day at school is nothing compared to a burned-over firefighter."

Riley continues talking about his own family. "You can't tell them. You have to show them, just like in the burn community. My kids will learn perspective in time. I'm not going to force it on them. They will be better people than me. I try to help them understand that their problems will pass. But the people I see often have a permanent loss. A 'change forever' empathy you either have or you learn."

Working towards one goal brought Dan's family together as they had never been before. Dan's family arrived on Saturday and Sunday and quickly teamed up with Jared of the Honor Guard. "We made a deal with the hospital that we could come to check, and the family would stay," he says. They also promised to follow all the protocols, and from the beginning, everyone in the room had to be covered from head to toe to protect Dan from infection.

Dan's brother Kelly, taller than Dan but just as lean and with a long beard, was first notified by their older sister Cindy the night of the burnover. When he heard the news at his home in Seattle, a flash of heat came over his body, and he had to sit down. He was especially alarmed when he heard Dan was on the flight to Utah. Kelly prayed, reaching out to his brother mentally, knowing he was about to experience misery.

Even before Marney died, Kelly knew his big brother had always been independent and disconnected from his family. Dan was stubborn about sharing information about himself, from grief to affection, and any loss of agency was at odds with who he was. Kelly prayed for a full hour, believing that "all paths lead to God." Then, with all plans in place, he was on the road to Salt Lake City.

When Kelly entered Dan's room, he had another hot flash and had to sit in the chair in the corner of the room for a moment. He had experience with patient advocacy, long-term hospital stays, and death. But seeing his big brother, who had always been the strong one, completely incapacitated, wrapped head to toe in gauze, was for a moment overwhelming.

Dan was barely lucid for the first couple of days as he fought the sedation and the oxygen. He knew where he was and that Kelly was there, but he was crashing. "Several times that first day, Dan checked out, coded out, and made the machines scream," said Kelly. "He would overbreathe against the oxygen. He fought against the entire system."

Behind the bed in the ICU room was a wall covered in vacuum and oxygen ports, all of which were constantly used by the firefighter. The monitor included blood pressure, oxygen level, respiration, and pulse recordings. At one point, every port in the wall was in use.

Kelly absorbed every ounce of discomfort that he saw in Dan. "He was very much not happy. He knew he was screwed. That was the best way to put it." Kelly knew all his strength, faith, and experience were required to help save Dan's life. He was determined to be a worthy fighter because his brother had always been one for him.

Starting the night he arrived, it was a game of how sedated they could keep him. Dan had three major surgeries to remove dead skin, using temporary cadaver skin. He was one of the Utah Center's sicker patients with Acute Respiratory Distress Syndrome (ARDS). The combination of the burns and his surgeries stressed his internal organs, most profoundly his lungs, which meant he had to be sedated, propelling him into delirium and incoherence. The next step was to induce a coma that would last twenty-four days. Even then, he had to be restrained. Everyone was determined to help Dan fight for his life. They worried from one day to the next if he were going to survive.

Hannah's brother, Will, sat in a chair against the wall, trying to absorb the shock of seeing his dad. When Hannah called him, he was in Columbia, Missouri, and hadn't seen Dan for years. They had just stopped effectively communicating. As he held his father's hand, Will cried. The idea of losing him, just seeing what he was going through, was too painful. He didn't want Dan suffering. To see him impossibly wounded was almost unbearable.

Will just wanted him to come out of the coma so they could communicate better. They'd had problems in the past, but they could try again. This was not how it was going to end. "Dad is one tough son of a bitch," Will says. They would get through this.

Then Dan died.

Let Him Go

"Stop torturing him!" Kelly screamed at the medical team. Dan had coded, and they were trying desperately to keep him going. The commotion of resuscitating him was a calamity, especially with the patient's brother pacing around the room, yelling at the doctors and nurses.

"Clear!" shouted an ICU doctor before he pressed the defibrillator paddles to the patient's chest. A nurse stepped in to do chest compressions, and another tried to get Kelly out of the way.

But Kelly had been around enough medical emergencies to know that the coma often plays with fire. Dealing with this kind of crisis was a delicate dance, one that often ends in a life lost. He watched Dan's battered body shock into the air and people pushing on his chest. Kelly believed that his brother had suffered enough.

"Let him go!"

Finally, the medical team kicked him out of the room, threatening to bring in security. Kelly left but continued to worry because he knew there was a Do Not Resuscitate order (DNR). Dan was adamant that he did not want to live as a vegetable. But no one had a copy of it. They brought him back twice when Kelly was there, and the expectations of success were never high.

But Dan kept coming back. Later, he said he did not want to, and it would have been easier to die. But he had to admit, "Sadly, my nature would not allow that." This feeling expressed the depth of torment to come.

Kelly had fought the team trying to resuscitate, but he was glad when Dan's heart was beating again. "I'm just grateful he did not lose at this dance."

Both Mandy and Margot were there one of the times Dan coded, with too many alarms sounding notes on a scale in disharmony, screaming. Mandy stopped breathing as they rushed her from the room. As an army of medical personnel attacked Dan in his bed, Margot hugged the hallway wall, trying to calm her anxiety. "It was scary. It all happened fast. I'm not sure we knew what was happening." It took fifteen minutes to get him back. The doctors could keep him alive but not bring Dan out of the coma. His oxygen was too low.

Even though the firefighter was out of danger for the moment, no one felt safe leaving him. "My dad was always this stud—a cool guy. A firefighter and skydiver," says Hannah. "But now I was afraid to leave him. They kept trying different antibiotics and different painkillers. Anything to help make it safe to bring him out of the coma."

Hannah kept waiting for the oxygen levels to reach a certain number. Every day, they would test, and she would anxiously wait. "Is his oxygen level good today?"

"Not yet."

Hannah was torn apart every time she needed to return to see her family in Ohio. Crying on the way to the airport, her heart raced with anxiety as she wondered if she would ever see him again. But she had to believe he would live. The alternative was too painful to contemplate.

Margot says the only consolation for everyone was how they all came together to become the family Dan needed them to be. They set up schedules and took turns from the beginning so he would never be alone. They talked to him as much as possible. They helped manage his care and stayed with the doctors and the nurses. They got him anything he needed at the hospital.

Dan was unaware of the incredible support and all the people there just for him. The small waiting room was not big enough for all the family members, the firefighters flying in from Red Lodge, and the Honor Guard.

"There were so many people," said Mandy. "He was asleep, but there was no peace around him because there was so much love from so many people. It was overwhelming all the time."

The waiting room was a hallway outside the ICU burn unit with about a dozen straight-back gray chairs. Four were connected into two seats without arms so that someone could put their head down on one, legs up on the other, curl tightly in a ball, and try to sleep. Dan's family and firefighters took every seat.

Usually, the Honor Guard only stays until the end, but Dan didn't die. "We sat in the waiting room. We had to walk through construction and COVID restrictions, so getting into the burn center was almost a no-go. Almost two years into COVID, the staff didn't like people encroaching on their space. It was huge that they let us in and on full guard duty all day Saturday. Nothing was going to stop us. But the hospital would not let us stay in the hall, so we went to the waiting room," says Jared.

The other patients' families saw the disparity with how Dan could have so many visitors. The Honor Guard could be intimidating or ominous. Eventually, there was an understanding that the uniformed presence was there as respect for the firefighter.

The Lovely Honor Guard

The firefighting family is made whole by the Honor Guard, who restore grace and pay respect to those who have left us.

Captain Anthony Widdison, sometimes called Wood, leaned on them more than he ever thought he would in 2018. It was then that he truly understood the significance of the Honor Guard.

The Mendocino Complex Fire was burning strong in Northern California, consuming half a million acres.[1] It raged for months with hundreds of firefighters assigned, including Utah's Assistant Chief Riley Pilgrim and Chief Matt Burchett. They were Utah's task force leaders, each managing thirty firefighters, working one shift off and on.

"I was off, and I got a call that we had an accident for a firefighter and that life support was flying to the hospital," says Riley. "In my head, I'm thinking, who could it be?" He considered all thirty men and narrowed it down to four possible firefighters: friends who were too painful to contemplate losing, including the youngest guy on his team. Deep in his gut, he knew something terrible had happened. Riley was racing in his truck, a minute behind the helicopter that took the firefighter to the closest semblance of an emergency room.

Riley entered a small medical facility and saw a nurse giving CPR to his firefighter, anxiously looking at the face. There was Matt. *It couldn't be Matt.* Riley stood at the foot of the bed that took up most of the facility's space and realized the other chief, responsible with him for the sixty firefighters, didn't have a mark on him. The injury was hidden deep inside. The nurse looked at Riley with no expression. There was nothing they could do.

The assistant chief watched the medical staff try valiantly with limited equipment. Until they stopped. The doctor looked up at him, saying nothing. Riley knew that Matt was gone. "When he looked at me, that was it." Riley was stunned, unable to move.

He wanted to lose himself in his grief but had no time. He was now responsible for sixty firefighters, all away from home, knowing that one of their own had been critically flown off the mountain. He had to call Matt's brothers. And he had to tell Anthony.

Riley says, "First, let me say that Cal Fire is the most professional, courteous, and thoughtful organization—no one is better. It was their fourth fatality that year." As the Utah team was coming off the mountain, he called his chief (Dan Petersen) and then called Dusty.

"I can't do it. It's too hard. Please call Wood for me," he said.

Silence was on the other end of the line for about ten seconds.

"All right."

When Riley told him about Matt's death, Assistant Chief Dusty Dern was on a fire in Utah.

"It was super, super shitty news. Matt was my first crew boss as a wildland firefighter. We also ski-patrolled together." Riley was overwhelmed, so Dusty started calling people on the list. But calling Anthony was about the worst duty he had ever had. The only way he knew how to do it was to be direct.

"Hey Anthony, Riley just called; Matt was killed in a fire in California." He heard the phone clatter to the floor as Anthony screamed. He couldn't stop cursing and yelling. Dusty held on to the call. He wasn't going to let go of the phone or Anthony.

It was all a blur for the Utah firefighters close to Matt. Their "blubbering" emotions made it impossible to think or function. After that death, that horrific event, they realized that effectively managing these tragedies required someone with an emotional degree of separation. They didn't realize that someone would soon come in full dress uniform.

Anthony says, "We were overwhelmed, lost in a fog when it was someone close to us. It still hurts."

By then, all sixty firefighters were in front of Riley. "I tell them straight. Matt passed away," he says. "We were in denial, shocked, and sad. It was so fresh in our minds."

Riley had no clue how to get Matt to a mortuary, bring him home, or contact his wife Heather, who was traveling, and his brother

Dominic. "I felt alone. Another guy and I were trying to navigate Matt from the hospital to the medical examiner to the funeral home and then transport family here and Matt home," says Riley.

Utah State didn't know what to do, even though the Utah firefighters had an agreement with the officials there and had connections to high-level people just two below the governor. Riley said, "We were fucked. They couldn't help us. We slept in the hospital, got Matt to the funeral home, and sent the sixty to get sleep, food, and shower."

Then, before he knew it, Cal Fire pulled out the stops with their Honor Guard already at the funeral home. Cal Fire personnel traveled from all over California and never left Matt's side, taking him home to Utah. "Within no time, the California governor gave his private airplane to pick up Matt's wife, brother, and Wood. Cal Fire flew Matt back to Utah in a C-130."

Chief Bruchette's casket, draped in the stars and stripes, was silently carried from the massive plane by the California Honor Guard. His brother, widow, and best friends followed solemnly behind. The chief's helmet would be presented to Heather. The bell would be rung nine times. The piper played "Amazing Grace." Matt was called home with one last page.

Anthony was incredibly grateful to California's elite officers for giving Matt the honor and grace he deserved. Not only did Matt deserve it, his brothers desperately needed to witness it. "Matt was my best friend. Having the Honor Guard protecting him and standing with him meant everything to me. He deserved the respect they were giving him. I know desperation and hopelessness."

Riley says, "We did not have these resources in Utah. Well, no more. We fixed it when we got back from California. We are doing this from now on. Jared is the one who makes it happen."

The Utah Fire Authority learned firsthand what Red Lodge Fire Rescue and fire departments everywhere suffered. With the Utah Burn

Center in their home, they initiated a world-class Honor Guard to support firefighters everywhere. Anthony said, "Without question, we can do a lot for these guys. We felt so helpless with Matt. We could imagine how they felt about Dan and being so far away."

Salt Lake Unified Fire Authority Is Family

Riley told Will and Tom that night in the cafeteria that even though UFA couldn't be there for eight months, they could fill the holes. Riley first told them to be prepared for the overwhelming support given to injured firefighters, have a point person, and send everything to that person, who was Sarah.

The Honor Guard was on duty in Utah in 2021 for Dan and his family. The officers were there to transport them wherever needed, and Jared brought them to dinner at the firehouse. "We facilitated what they were about to see," says Riley. "At first, we were concerned we were bringing family members together that weren't very close. That is why we got Layne in there. In the end, we felt very close to all of them."

It is the job of the Honor Guard to give back to those who came before. Riley says, "Any firefighter from any department, we will honor them at their funeral. We'll guard the casket and fold the flag." A firefighter killed in the line of duty is more in-depth. For the family, sometimes the Honor Guard is the only look into the firefighting service, and they make their lives a little bit easier with a glimpse of hope and light. They help them through the funeral process, or, as with Dan, they stand guard at their door, hoping they get better. Dan was one of the few with such extensive injuries who survived.

"The team stepped up," says Petersen. "I just ensured they had the resources they needed. Honor Guard presence provides honor to the family, but we don't want to be intrusive. It was very unique for Dan to live. Or for the Honor Guard to be involved for that long. The Honor Guard ensures the family knows how respected the person is because of their chosen profession. It's not often that we get to stay to help survivors."

Throughout the following month, the family and the firefighters from Red Lodge took turns visiting. When one person left, another person took over. They wanted Dan to always sense they were there, as evidenced by the dozens of masks, disposable gowns, boots, hats, and gloves thrown out daily. Family bonds could not have been stronger, nor could their bond with the UFA firefighters and the firefighters coming back and forth from Montana.

According to Kordenbrok for the *Billings Gazette*, "Red Lodge Fire Rescue [was] continuing to coordinate visits to Steffensen, something that is complicated in part by the busy fire season in Carbon County. Additionally, Hyfield said they don't want to overwhelm him, his family, or the hospital, by sending too many people at once. 'He's got a special place in all of our hearts and I think it's important that we have somebody there that's with him while he's undergoing his surgeries,' Hyfield said."[2]

Red Lodge Fire Rescue fought fires, searched for Tate, and supported Dan as he lay in a coma. Still, they were about to find out how much worse the summer would get.

CHAPTER ELEVEN

The Summer of Hell

As prayers rose above the Beartooth Mountains and found their way to Dan, still in a coma at the University of Utah Burn Center, the search continued for the missing hiker. The wilderness silence was haunted by the helicopter rotors lifting daily to search for Tate. The entire town was on a first-name basis with Tate because her family called her Tate. "Will we find Tate today?"

The firefighters' ire was high as the Robertson Draw Fire continued to burn. Even though it was contained, every small smoke or flame flare would cause panic enough to send an engine to check it out.

The town leaned on each other and their gods. They added Tate and her family to their prayers for Dan, for him to wake up and heal, to get past the terrible ordeal of surviving his burns, and to come home.

Broadway was paved with bleakness. Walking down the historic Western main street, every once in a while, a person would stop in the middle of the sidewalk and shed a tear. The valley's atmosphere was sad, quiet, and spiritual. No one thought it could get any worse in Red Lodge, Montana, a town accurately described with one word—heart.

It would soon break into unimaginable grief. Ryan Ples was a qualified engine boss and participant on Red Lodge Fire Rescue's fuel mitigation crew and was one of Tom's valued restaurant employees. When Ryan wasn't in the restaurant or fighting fires, he was always on the ski mountain, working or playing in some capacity. Ryan's wife Bonnie was the general manager at the restaurants.

They and their children, as well as Tom, his wife, and their two daughters, are among the many families that made Red Lodge home. Their lives could have been photographed for a Montana magazine.

Ryan was the one always lying back in the chair with a grin on his face and a great attitude. No one could imagine that this very talented athlete and master of the outdoors, Ryan, could fall on his skateboard and crack his skull on the pavement.

The night sky was dark, with clouds hiding the stars, and Ruth was finally asleep, her mind at rest from the eventful days. It took several calls, several rings, to wake her up. When she finally answered groggily, she realized it was Jon calling from the hospital.

"You need to come to be with Bonnie. Now," he said. Jon was always in control and usually betrayed little emotion, but he broke down on the phone. He could do that with Ruth. Seeing the damage to Ryan's head, he was afraid a brother firefighter was most likely going to leave behind his beautiful young wife and children.

Ruth was his first call. They had worked together for years. They trust each other the same way Ruth and Sarah do. It was a gut punch for Ruth. But she was the shoulder-in-chief for everyone in the firehouse. According to Sarah, Ruth makes a nest for anyone in the community needing to be safe.

Being strong and handling crises was just what Ruth did, especially for families. Bonnie and Ryan were as much her family as anyone's. Her daughters and the Ples kids were on the Nordic ski team together. Ryan was the president of the Firefighters Association. Ruth and Bonnie saw each other almost every day.

Tom was realistic about Ryan's condition. He met Ruth at the hospital with his shoulders hanging lower and lower and told her to clear her schedule. "Your only responsibility is Bonnie and her family." Bonnie leaned on Ruth's shoulder, arms wrapped tightly, bawling uncontrollably. Ryan stayed on life support as his and Bonnie's families arrived in Red Lodge.

Tears ran down Tom's face many times. Amy says, "He needed to cry. It was good to show emotion to everyone. He did his job, but with tears."

One of Ryan's best friends, Lieutenant Amy Hyfield, dealt with the emergency as if in a fog. She says, "I didn't answer the page right away. I didn't know it was Ryan." She took on the communication duty for Tom. Her focus on the job was her way to cope with the personal pain of losing her close colleague and friend.

At the same time, chaos and engines were blasting loudly in the town. Dan was in a coma in Utah, Ryan was on life support, and Tate was still missing as the annual Harley Davidson rally roared up and down Broadway. Helicopters were still flying overhead, searching for Tate. Experienced hikers traversed five possible peaks, asking themselves, "Where would you go? Which mountain would you take? What would be your path?"

Every air and ground resource was there. They had finally realized it was a recovery effort, not a rescue effort. Conversations all over town were speculation. Did a bear get her? Where would it have dragged her body? Tate was no longer a name but an emotion.

Tom's priority was a twenty-four-hour command center that never closed. His leadership never faltered, but his feelings were raw. Tate was about the same age as his daughters. Ryan was his long-time employee. Dan was still touch and go. The chief would walk around daily with tears in his eyes as he answered questions from the anxious people in his town.

Before she was in charge of being with Bonnie, Ruth would meet the rescuers coming back down from the mountain, always with water and granolas. Each time, they walked the path they were assigned and on each return she could see the disappointment on their faces. They had not found Tate.

There was a morbid tension throughout town as Ryan remained on life support. Every day, there were tests on Ryan's brain. Every day, helicopters were searching for Tate. Every day, there were prayers for Dan to live. Finally, the tests showed Ryan wasn't there anymore. On August 11, Lieutenant Ryan Ples was pronounced dead.

The ski mountain above the town was drenched with light. Several shades of green blanketed the slope as the towering lifts stood silent. The August sun was a welcome relief to the dark mood throughout the valley. Hundreds gathered for a firefighter's funeral for Ryan Ples. Captain Will Bernard returned home from managing another fire.

Speaking at the service, Will said, "When Ryan joined our department, neither he nor his family understood they were joining another family. His family is here. We are here in the good and the tough times."

Tyler read words of an unknown origin that Hank had found posted on Ryan's board:

Every sixty seconds you spend angry, upset, or mad is a full minute of happiness you will never get back.

Life is short. Break the rules.

Forgive quickly. Kiss slowly. Love truly. Laugh uncontrollably. And never regret anything that made you smile.

These were words Ryan carried with him during his short life.

Firefighters saluted as they gave Bonnie the Stars and Stripes and Ryan's helmet. Nine bells rang out and echoed up every canyon carved in the Beartooth Mountains, followed by the ghost of the sound of piper Brad Logan playing "Amazing Grace." Finally, there was a last page for firefighter Ryan Ples. He was called to duty one last time. The final page said, "He was called home to the arms of the Lord."

That page, that moment was when Lieutenant Hyfield let go of her duty in public relations. Amy knew her dear friend was gone and cried.

On August 21, hikers found Tate's foot sticking out of the ground. She had died from a rockslide on the first day of her hike. Her remains were retrieved by a helicopter the following morning. SAR thought she left her tent to summit a 12,000-foot peak. "Tate was a fiercely independent, adventurous soul who loved the mountains," the family said in a statement. "We find some solace in knowing she passed in a place she loved."[1]

Lieutenant Hyflied says, "As a team, we eventually knew we were not looking for a live person. What else could we have done? There was a lot of that kind of uncertainty that existed then. I was questioning whether we did everything we could to find her. Was she alive for a while?"

Ivan Kosorok, who had first found her tent, helped with the recovery. Ruth knows him as a friend of her son Sean's from junior high. She says, "I know picking up the pieces was hard for him. No matter how strong or kind a man a mountain man is. That is still a tough thing to do."

Everyone in town still grappled with dreadful emotions about Dan and Ryan Ples as part of the Red Lodge Fire Rescue family. Recalling tragedies in detail can wound even the most seasoned medical and fire personnel—the blood in the street for Jon, Ivan recovering Tate, and the horrible things happening to Dan in Utah.

Red Lodge Fire Rescue team members were doing their best to support the people in need: Dan's family, Ryan's family, and Tatum Morrell's family. But the first responders were also struggling. It was time to take up Utah's Chief Petersen's offer of support and call in Layne.

The behavioral specialist fell in love with the town because of its unity. "I've seen a lot of small towns but never one like this. They all look out for each other." Thanks to their cohesion, Layne could speed up the process. The firefighter family and blood family are one and the same. It makes it easier for them to emote and cry with each other.

Danny says, "It was good to know this isn't just one of us. We all needed counseling. We were not dealing with this. It's hard to admit when you're not bulletproof. It's hard to admit how much this hurt."

But firefighters are not good communicators. There was recovering to do, and none had training in psychology. Layne encouraged them to discuss the trauma with each other. The town needed to open up to each other to get in touch with their feelings.

Layne says, "It wasn't hard because it was already that kind of town."

Layne explained that first responders deal with trauma stressors differently than an average citizen—even different from the military. The most important thing to set up is a peer group.

Danny says, "There was a heck of a turnout with Layne for the peer groups. We were on that call too. It's shit. So let's talk about it."

"Fourteen took advantage of the individual sessions, and everyone stood out as people caring about each other. In these sessions, the concern for Dan was paralyzing," says Layne. People were scrambling to take care of his lawn or pick up his mail. They needed something to do to make a difference.

Layne always asked, "What would Dan want you to do?

Layne says it was easy to answer. Dan would like everyone to train more.

UFA Chief Dan Petersen asked Layne to become a full-time therapist in 2019, not long after they set up their Honor Guard system after the death of Chief Matt Burchett in California. Layne is still a firefighter, paramedic, and Hazmat tech.

The International Association of Firefighters (IAFF) found that firefighters don't seek out help for mental issues because of the stigma that says they can't be weak. They can't have problems. They are the ones who solve problems. There is also a vulnerability issue. Firefighters don't like to be or appear vulnerable.

After 9/11, expectations changed. Firefighters became "America's bravest." Fighting fires used to be just a really good blue-collar job. Now it is: Who is your hero? Batman, Superman, Fireman. The otherworldly expectations are something that nobody can meet. They have to be the bravest they can be and can't admit they hurt, let alone that they don't feel safe.

"The town did not like feeling vulnerable. That is the first thing we worked on," Layne says. Peer support was a national initiative, but it was new or emerging in Red Lodge, where everything was terrible that summer. They were able to do it quickly and well because of the bond and the love they already had.

Most therapists don't understand the upside-down lives resulting from a firefighter's schedule. They are on call all the time. They know they are going to go to work every day. They can't turn it off. Normal therapy techniques don't work as well.

With first responders, it is important to understand that guilt is a by-product of the job. It is ever present because taking responsibility for the scene doesn't always work out how they want it to. Everyone is guaranteed to die sometime, so first responders feel they are fighting a losing battle. The sense of responsibility can be overwhelming.

Layne says, "We are not suicidal. We have come to grips with the job, but it is still tough for everyone to grieve. The main feelings are anger, frustration, and anxiety, but it comes down to worry and love. Everyone felt helpless."

When emotions come, good or bad, they are good. A firefighter needs to know emotions will change. Eating, sleeping, and drinking water are essential. Anxiety and worry stop people from sleeping, making them prone to behavioral health issues. A person's ability to manage stress deteriorates without sleep. If people keep their feelings bottled up, they will explode, as some members of Red Lodge Fire Rescue did that summer.

"Think of it as physics," Layne says. "Energy can only be moved, manipulated, or used, not created or destroyed. Those feelings are energy. They will exceed the container it is in. It will come out in blow-ups, alcohol, or suicide. Move the energy by talking."

Everyone in Red Lodge started talking, leaning on each other, and praying. One community member said she had to find out if Dan was still alive every morning. Until she knew his status, she couldn't breathe.

Another community member reached out to Dan spiritually, as if it were a one-on-one conversation, calling out to him from miles away, "If you are willing to come back, we're here. We want you to come home. Come home if you can get through this and do what it takes. If it's too hard and you can't come back, okay, but we are here if you choose to come back."

The universe was listening. Dan was coming out of his coma. Dan's son sat beside his bed in the chair. Dan opened his eyes and didn't recognize him. He even asked, "Who the hell are you?"

When Dan finally recognized his son Will after so many years apart, his tears were uncontrollable. When he first came out of the coma, Dan was physically and mentally unstable. He was not fully awake or aware for another two weeks. He was very emotional and heavily medicated. About the same time Tate was found, Dan began to be mindful of the tremendous work ahead of him.

His recovery and Red Lodge's recovery were parallel.

CHAPTER TWELVE

Horrible Things

DAN LAY IN A HOSPITAL BED WITH HIS BURNED BODY SHROUDED IN gauze to keep the outside world from disturbing the progress of his skin grafts and wound care. He thought about Tyler and Will, the men who trained and mentored him. His emotions were a kaleidoscope turning in his brain—shame, regret, and failure, unable to discern a pattern with any sense. He knew they had visited. Everyone had seen him small.

Looking down at the IV stuck in his arm, pumping pain meds that barely took the edge off, he wondered if any of this was worth it. To awaken from a coma wasn't just a mental ordeal. Dan's physical reality was horrible and humiliating.

Even basic COVID protocols became an issue for him, not just because they reminded him of when Marney died.

"Dan, you have to wear your mask," nurses would tell him whenever they entered his room.

"I don't have any ears," Dan said. How was he supposed to wear a mask without ears?

Margot was there right after they brought him out of the coma. "He was aware that he was burned. He was extremely confused, didn't know where or why he was there, and couldn't remember his address."

Dan was independent and didn't need anyone. He had always been good at pushing people out of his life. Lying in a hospital bed with people taking care of him, pitying him, went against his very core.

"He was angry," says Mandy. "He didn't want to be in that situation at all. I'm not sure he wanted to live. He's a pretty determined guy. He didn't understand that we would have been very sad if he died."

Coming out of a coma is not like a light switch you can turn on and off. Medication slowly lets patients process everything independently. This helps keep them calm to get a good night's rest until they know where they are, explains Erik. "Then they forget and start all over, slowly bringing down the ventilation and the meds to allow them to sort of sober up."

The difficult and important part is that everyone has to do their job. "PT has to move the patient's arms," Erik says. "Every person on the unit's job is helping him process that he is waking up and realizing where he is. Family being there is essential. Imagine having a stranger tell you. It's much better if it comes from a voice you recognize. It's a world of difference for a patient."

Face care was especially critical because it had so much to do with morale. "A lot of care to the face," says Erik. "I found a central aspect is for them to see their face. It helps them realize they will heal. They see themselves in the mirror and think, 'Cool, I can heal from this.'"

But Dan refused to look in the mirror for two weeks after waking from the coma. So, one day, Erik grabbed a razor.

"What the hell?" said Dan, unable to use his hands to protect his face, turning his head awkwardly back against his pillow, stretching his neck, and grimacing. He hadn't yet realized how much his face had healed.

"Dan, are you fucking kidding me? I'm going to shave your face now," insisted Erik.

Dan finally laid back in resignation. "In that case, I want my mustache back."

"I know it's a fucking rocking mustache, but you can't start growing it yet."

Waking from the coma was like walking out of a fog. Dan had nightmares; all of them involved not being able to move. Once, he dreamed he was stuck in the corner of the room. Another time, he kept looking at a vista of sand and hills in the immense desert. The sky was hazy, but the sun was blazing like a fire. He just knew he had to cross it.

In another dream, he was in a houseboat that had flipped over in the water and he had to get out, but again, he could not move. He also remembered a dream in which he was stuck in an old mental hospital on top of a mountain peak, unable to escape. He was trying to get down a long snaking ramp that went on forever. The ramp was the way out of the coma, and his brother Kelly was waiting for him at the end. The dreams were vivid and unsettling.

All told, Dan had eighteen surgeries. He had received skin grafts on his arms, hands, face, back, abdomen, and both of his legs. Dr. Callie Thompson, a young, outgoing brunette with a voice that exuded confidence and friendliness, knew the importance of skin repair. She had dedicated her life to burn survivors and wanted Dan to survive and thrive after his injury.

"I can fix it," she said. "Once I don't have to worry about you dying, we can work on stuff."

Most of Dan's surgeries were in the first two days or soon after he was induced into a coma.

When he was out of the coma, his back was healed, allowing him to lie down. They used Dan's own healthy skin for the grafts in what's called an autograft procedure, mainly from his belly, back, or lower thigh, to cover the larger areas that were burned. Skin was taken from his collarbone and groin area for the intense burns. Not enough was available for all of his burns, so allograft, or cadaver skin, had to be used to temporize the areas that weren't yet grafted while he grew new skin for more autografts.

A composite graft was necessary to replace Dan's ears with skin and cartilage. Both cadaver skin and Dan's chest and abdomen provided the donor skin for his ears. The doctors poked holes into the healthy skin, also called meshing, to stretch the skin over a larger area to help it heal, and then secured it with staples and dressing. The donor site heals after surgery but often takes longer than the graft site. Some of Dan's skin grafts didn't take the first time because of infection or bleeding and had to be redone.

After the surgeries, wound care and physical therapy, or PT, which began right when he woke up, were agonizing for Dan. The arm burns were sore as hell and were popping open and tearing blisters. Donor sites always have the worst nerve pain. Wound care came first, and the word terrible is not enough to describe it. Afterward, a sponge bath gets some dead skin off, which also really hurts. Two more PT sessions followed.

The best donor site is fresh skin that has never been taken to increase the likelihood that it will heal faster. Because of the depth of the burns, the superficial veins that run under the skin were also damaged and had to be excised. These veins are responsible for the vast majority of the blood that returns to the heart. Deep veins must compensate, and they are never again one hundred percent effective, resulting in more swollen legs. Dan could wear compression socks or sit with his legs raised, but that would just be a reminder that he was hurt, so he didn't want to do that. This was an example of his stubbornness.

"To this day, my elbows, fingers, and knees all need stretching," he says. "My thumb to the little finger. Nerves are gone in the skin. People don't understand it is a lifelong maintenance of skin. Without stretching and Vaseline, the skin would pull back on my wrists, hands, knees, and elbows mainly. My face would be crazy tight. It's hard to whistle and smile. My lips are always chapped or numb. My ears and lips feel like frostbite. I must be conscious when eating if something is hanging out of my mouth, like going to the dentist."

Between the pain and anguish, Dan leaned on friends. "I don't think I can get through this," he said on a call to Dr. Brad Fouts back in Red Lodge.

His friend knew it would not be easy, but he also knew Dan and the words that would motivate him. He had to remind him that he was strong. "Dan, you also need to consider that you inspire the community, and we need one right now."

A week after Ryan Ples died, Assistant Chief Jim Avant visited Dan. He had been returning from Washington when he got the page that Dan had been burned. His pager would not stop beeping. He pulled over on the highway to get the news.

Burnover in Joliet

He turned the driving over to his family, and they got back in the car.

Then Tom called him and said, "It's Dan."

Jim felt pressure in his chest as grief grabbed hold of him. He cried as he told his family. The two friends had known each other since before Dan became a firefighter. They were neighbors. Jim knew Marney and had met Mandy and Margot.

When Jim visited Dan in Utah, he realized that Dan had yet to hear the news about Ryan Ples and wanted him to find out from one of the chief officers. He was prepared for Dan to be out of it. Jim waited in Dan's room as he returned from walking around the unit's floor. Jim could tell Dan was in a lot of pain but was very happy to see him.

Jim held his hand carefully and tried to reassure him. "Dan, I have something to tell you," he said quietly. "Ryan Ples was in a skateboard accident. He cracked his skull and died."

Dan grabbed Jim's arm as he sat on his bed. He said nothing as he cried. And Jim cried with him. "I just don't know if this is worth it. It is so hard," Dan sobbed.

Jim said, "Dan, there will always be a place for you at the station. We need you."

Dan had lived for the Red Lodge Fire Rescue. Jim wanted to encourage him because he was struggling. Dan was glad that Jim came but was getting tired. He was quiet.

Finally, Jim said, "We can't wait for you to come home." Dan was heavily medicated. Jim could tell that everything on him was hurting.

Tim arrived that same day and worked closely with Kelly on medical and financial updates. "They were doing horrible things to Dan. I would tell him details one day and then repeat them the next to see if he remembered them." Tim was also on the phone daily with Mike Sell, the Montana State Fund workers' compensation agent who was acutely in tune with Dan's condition and progress. Seeing the cost of every surgery, every moment of therapy, and wound care, Mike was impressed with Dan's tenacity. "Jeez, he must be a tough old bastard," he told Tim.

Coping with Ryan's mortality was hard enough for Dan. Then he saw a post on September 5 from the Laurel Fire Department about Captain Sean McCleary:

Thoughts and prayers go out to our brother, Captain Sean McCleary of the Laurel Volunteer Fire Department. A glioblastoma tumor has been identified attached to his brain. He will have surgery Sunday morning to remove as much as they can. We love you, Sean, and our hearts and prayers go out to you, Kari, and the boys. We are all family.

On September 2, 2021, Sean's wife, Kari McCleary, got a phone call from her stepson Colton: "We just called an ambulance for Dad."

As reported to KTVQ news, Sean had been on a fire and recalled: "'I grabbed the radio and keyed dispatch, but when they answered, I didn't know what I was going to say,' Sean said. 'I had it all in my mind, but I couldn't say it. Thirty seconds later, I keyed the mic again, and the same thing happened. The third time, I started stuttering.'" Because of a large glioblastoma—a tumor—on his brain, Sean blacked out. He told KTVQ News, "I didn't know if I was going to wake back up."

The news was hard on Dan. He thought about how Sean and Ryan were younger than him, both with wives and children. Both were happy men. Sean was kind and always smiling. Ryan was laid back and always cheerful. They were so much different than him. He had to ask himself why two men, two brothers who were happy to be alive and surrounded by people who needed them, were dead or dying while he had survived to go through so much pain.

"What the hell is God thinking?"

CHAPTER THIRTEEN

"Let me die."

FRIENDS AND FAMILIES IN RED LODGE PRAYED FERVENTLY FOR A HERO to come home. Dan had sensed their petitions two states away while still in a coma.

"I heard them. A tingle in my brain called me to wake up and come home," he says. "Once I woke up, we had long conversations, me and God. Every day, I prayed, 'Don't let it hurt anymore.' We talked a lot about dying. I wanted to die, and why wasn't God just letting me die? It would be so much easier."

Dan turned the decision to live or die over to a power greater than himself. He resented, even hated, therapy so much that his anger was how he handled the intense physical pain and mental anguish. Resentment was a new dependency because, in wound care, the pain never stopped. The agony never stopped. He was literally losing himself, bit by bit.

They removed all the dead skin until they reached good skin. Morphine barely took the edge off the pain. Every session, Dan lay on a metal table, a cold hose on his body, as the water pooled under him before slushing down all the blood and pieces of flesh.

Dan says, "There are pieces of you going down the drain. Your body is going down the drain. I did not have any confidence that it would ever end."

Dan's request to God became even stronger, asking him to stop the pain. He could only see one way to accomplish this. "Let me die."

It wasn't an empty request: he wasn't afraid to die. Because of what had happened to Sean and Ryan, he was keenly aware of mortality.

Dan says, "I cried a lot."

Burn patients have all the right to be surly and uncooperative. In the beginning, Dan was one of the worst. As her first big burn patient, he was a challenge to Nurse Emily Pascua. The dark brunette can stand in the doorway and magically change the room's mood, and her patients start to heal from her smile, demeanor of hope, and compassion.

When she first saw him, she thought he would surely die due to the extent of his injuries. His unique ability to survive made her practically adopt him. Emily says, "Dan was the worst patient because he kept saying 'I'm fine' when he wasn't." At first, he resented being asked.

One time, Dan closed his eyes and ignored Emily.

Emily said, "Listen, Dan, you can have a ten-minute pity party. Now, let's get moving."

Dan didn't budge. He opened his eyes to glare at her from under his brow. She smiled and showed him her watch. The minutes were up. He got moving.

When he wasn't talking to God, he was talking and listening to Emily. She convinced him to do what the doctors told him to do, even though he hated it, in order to heal.

Dan's grumpiness was not reserved for her. He had impossible pain just using his hands or walking. He couldn't brush his teeth.

He said to Xavier, "Help me."

Xavier said, "Figure it out."

Dan appreciated this approach later.

Dan despised anything that made him feel hurt, including the braces at night that kept his arms straight. The night was already dark enough for his mood. The room smelled like medicine and machines. He was forced to sleep on his back, meaning he didn't sleep.

He told Xavier and Daphne, "I hate these braces. I'm not wearing them anymore."

"You don't need them," said Xavier, taking them off.

Dan protested to everyone. "I want to eat ice chips but can't reach my mouth." He started crying.

Emily helped him stand up and move away from the bed. He leaned on her shoulder, a tall man against a much smaller woman, and took small steps. Every day he took a few more. And then a few more until finally, leaning on Emily, he walked outside to breathe the fresh Utah air.

The hospital became Dan's home. He tried to focus on things outside of the pain, like the floor plan of his unit. He figured out that walking a mile took nineteen times around. For now, he was happy to complete one lap. On his first trips around the floor, he saw a lot of "littles," or kids aged six to nine, suffering from burn accidents.

Dan sensed the despair in the hospital rooms, knowing other patients were intubated on a ventilator like he had been. The most heart-breaking thing to see was a closed door to a patient's room. That usually meant the burn was serious, maybe even fatal. He could hear the sound of vacuum ports working on wounds, lungs, and throats. A toothbrush is driven by a vacuum port. Oxygen ports operate other mechanisms. Though despair was inside the rooms, hope was outside with the staff. Their job was to always enter a patient's room with a smile.

In the unit, other patients were led through the hallway, including children with horrible wounds. Dan was amazed by their calm demeanor of acceptance. The noise of other beds rolling into the surgical area broke the tension, only to fill it with dread. The big closed wooden doors with blinds shut, covering the glass, concealed the pain. In one corner of the floor was the PT room. Dan looked for inspiration in the people there, but they were struggling.

Dan says, "They were not doing shit. And I couldn't do shit. They were ahead of me in time, which was disappointing. If they can't, how will I?"

And after PT, there was more wound care. Dan says, "Every day. With God and morphine, I kept getting through it."

One day, a young pre-teen boy was sitting outside the PT room. His right arm, shoulder, and side of his neck were entirely burned from a Fourth of July accident twelve days before Dan had been burned. Dan found out the boy's name was Kevin.

At first, Kevin just turned his head and ignored him.

The following week, there was a nod. They made eye contact, and Dan saw the almost vacant expression of someone trying to forget they were in incredible pain and discomfort—something he was also trying to forget. He wondered if he had the same vacant stare.

"Good morning, Kevin." Dan thought he had to keep trying and did for several days.

Finally, days later, Kevin turned his head toward the tall man and said, "Hi." There was a tiny bit of gleam that had replaced the vacancy. Each day, the "hi" would grow a little more friendly.

Their times in therapy coincided, and Kevin and Dan could commiserate with just a look because they both hated PT. It took weeks to go from three-pound weights to five-pound. With burned hands, it was tough to even grip them.

Then, one day, Dan walked by Kevin's room, and the door was open. He stopped in the doorway and said, "Hi."

Kevin actually smiled back at him. "Hi."

The conversation expanded to a few more words about their burns, scars, and pain. But Dan never made it into the room despite fewer gown requirements.

The common touch points began with their skin grafts and pain. "We didn't dwell on it." Skin grafts don't grow with age. Kevin has to get them for the rest of his life. All the kids at burn camp have to go through it. That is why Dr. Thompson works so hard to get all the kids' surgeries early in the schedule—so they can swim in the pool at camp.

Kevin and Dan became a heartening sight walking the halls together—a 6'2" man and a small child. Words unspoken. The longer stride deliberately slowed to keep pace with the short.

Darlene Rawlin, Kevin's grandmother, says, "I remember the day Dan came into the hospital. I didn't know what happened; I just knew there were men in uniform standing by his door. As I walked by, I would always say hello. By then, Kevin was there for fifteen days, and then weeks went by, and they were in physical therapy. I got to know the wonderful person Dan is. Without Dan, Kevin would never make it through physical therapy."

Neither would Dan have made it without Kevin.

It would be even harder for Dan to attempt group therapy because it required emotional work. Besides, Dan couldn't sit in the chair in the corner long enough to use his iPad for the group. He could only sit up in bed, and he couldn't hear.

Dan says, "I didn't want to be in the group because I didn't want to be part of the dynamic of injured people." Group therapy was another area where he was stubborn. At first, he would not accept that his life had changed. Taking a new life inventory, self-searching, admitting shortcomings, and asking hard questions was always painful for Dan, who was already hurting.

Photo Gallery

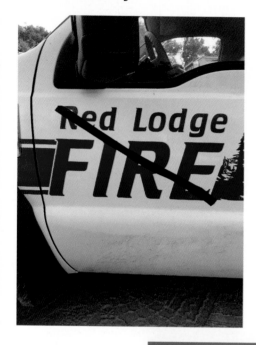

Engine marked with diagonal black tape after a firefighter fatality.[1] PHOTOGRAPH COURTESY OF DAN STEFFENSEN.

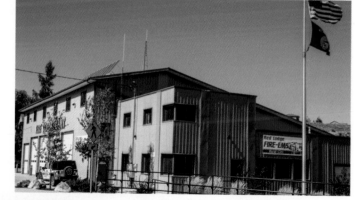

Red Lodge Fire Rescue. PHOTOGRAPH COURTESY OF RED LODGE FIRE RESCUE.

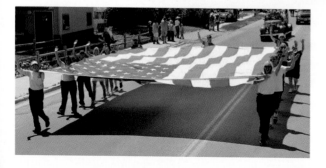

Red Lodge Fire Rescue carrying flag on Broadway in the July Fourth Parade. PHOTOGRAPH COURTESY OF RED LODGE FIRE RESCUE.

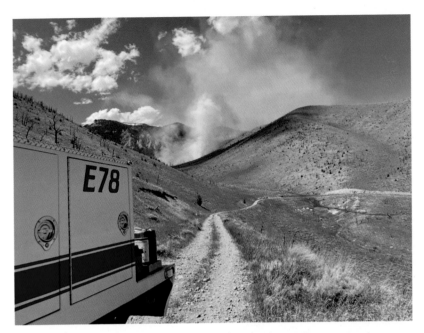

The beginning of the Robertson Draw Fire, "Dan's Engine 78." PHOTOGRAPH COUR-
TESY OF DAN STEFFENSEN.

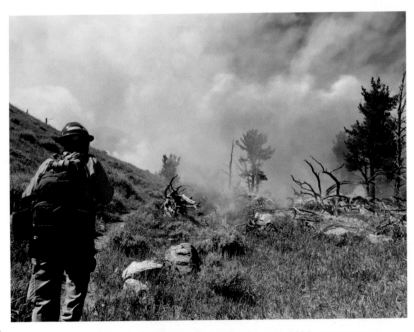

Getting a closer look at the Robertson Draw Fire, June 13, 2021. PHOTOGRAPH
COURTESY OF KATY HEDTKE.

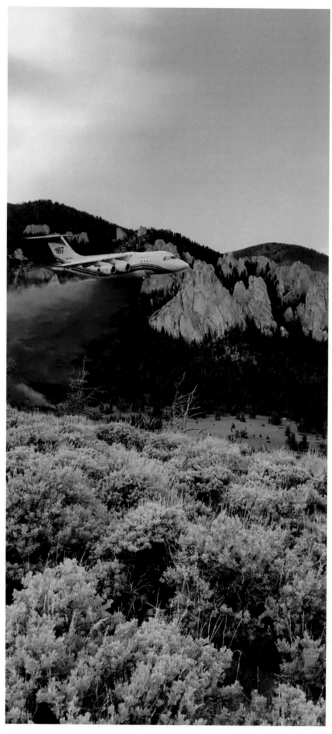

Dan directed the retardant drop for Robertson Draw Fire. PHOTO-
GRAPH COURTESY OF DAN STEFFENSEN.

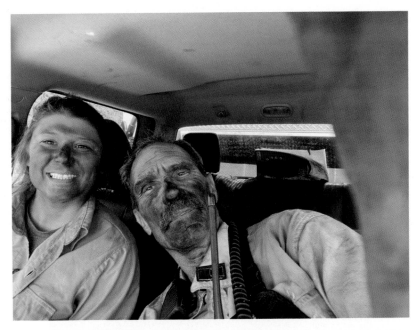

Katy Hedtke and Dan Steffensen, 2021. PHOTOGRAPH COURTESY OF DAN STEFFENSEN.

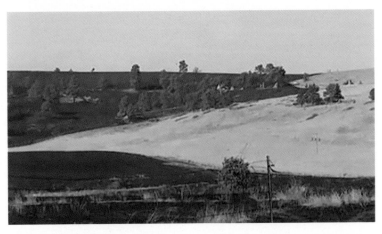

Harris Fire burnover on a bluff near Farewell Road. PHOTOGRAPH COURTESY OF RED LODGE FIRE RESCUE.

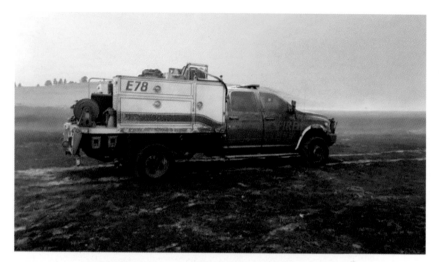

Engine 78 after Harris Fire Burnover. PHOTOGRAPH COURTESY OF RED LODGE FIRE RESCUE.

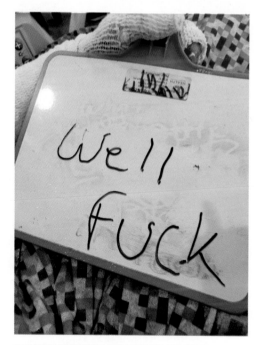

PHOTOGRAPH COURTESY OF WILL BERNARD.

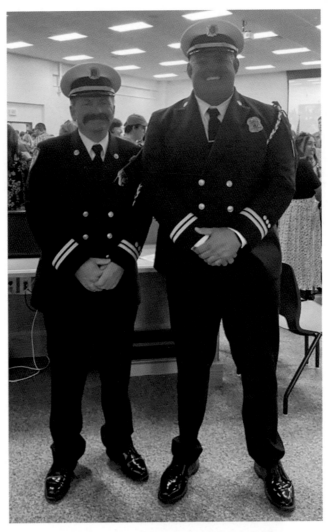

Honor Guard Captains Jared Wayman and Tommy Miller. PHOTO-
GRAPH COURTESY OF SALT LAKE UNIFIED FIRE AUTHORITY.

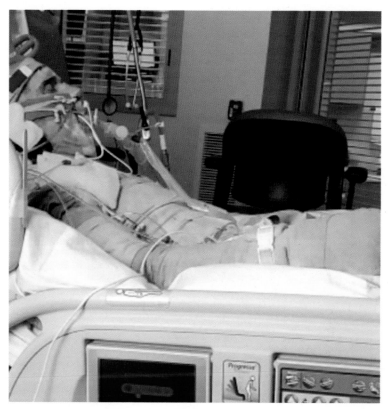

Dan lay in a coma for twenty-four days. PHOTOGRAPH CREDIT SUSIE STEFFENSEN.

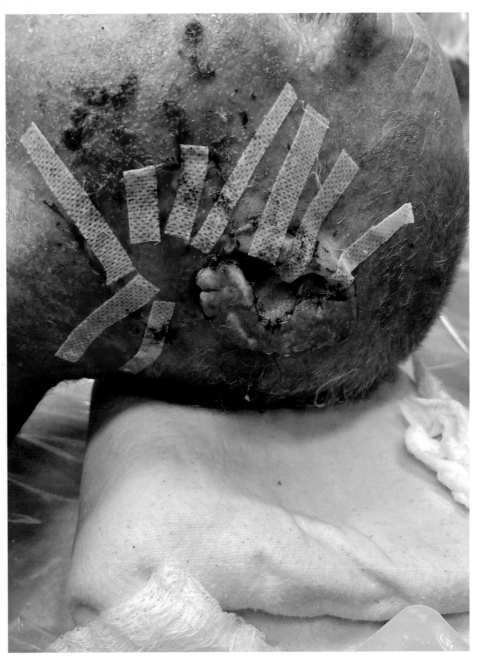

Dan needs both ears replaced. PHOTOGRAPH COURTESY OF KELLY STEFFENSEN.

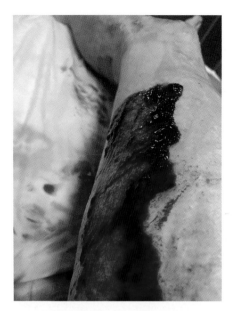

Donor skin site from Dan's leg. PHOTO-GRAPH COURTESY OF DAN STEFFENSEN.

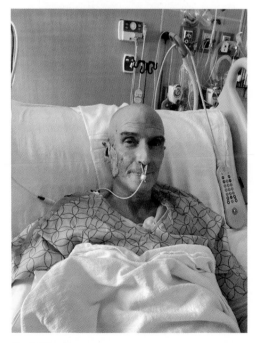

Dan's New Ear. PHOTOGRAPH COURTESY OF KELLY STEFFENSEN.

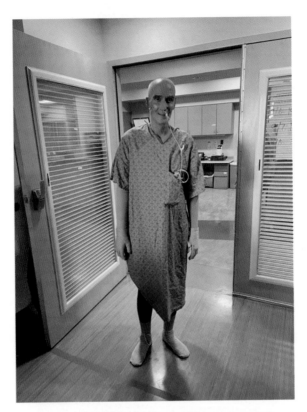

Dan recovered in Salt Lake City in 2021. PHOTOGRAPH
COURTESY OF KELLY STEFFENSEN.

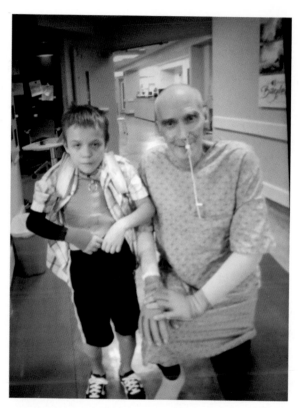

Dan and Kevin. PHOTOGRAPH COURTESY OF KELLY STEFFENSEN.

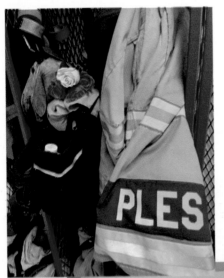

Flowers placed in Ryan Ples' Locker.
PHOTOGRAPH COURTESY OF RED LODGE
FIRE RESCUE.

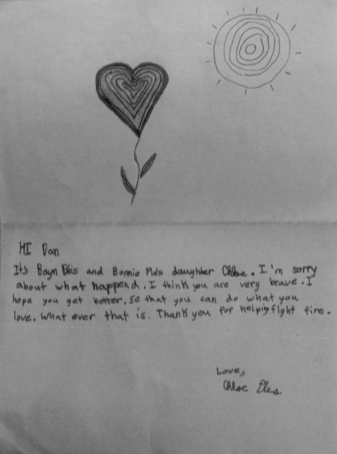

HI Dan

It's Rayn Ples and Bonnie Ples daughter Chloe. I'm sorry about what happend. I think you are very brave. I hope you get better, so that you can do what you love. what ever that is. Thank you for helpiy fight fire.

Love,
Chloe Ples

Chloe Ples Letter. PHOTOGRAPH COURTESY OF DAN STEFFENSEN.

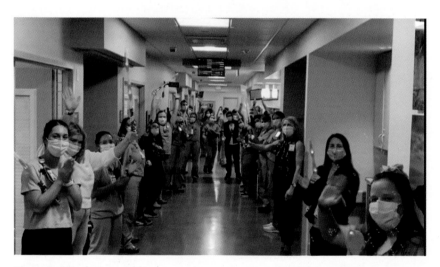

The end of Dan's Tunnel of Love. PHOTOGRAPH COURTESY OF DOUG BUDGE.

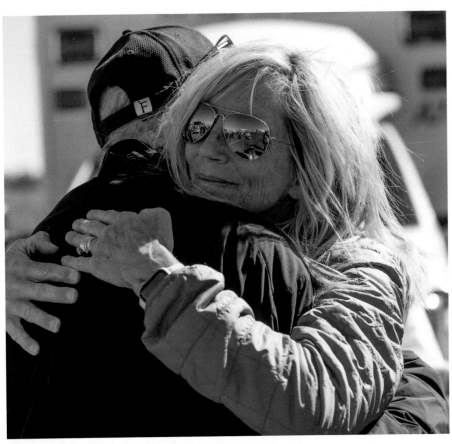

Sarah Ewald welcomes Dan home at Red Lodge Airport. PHOTOGRAPH COURTESY OF COLLEEN KILBANE.

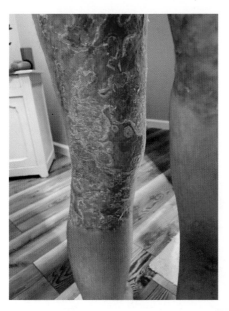

Dan's left leg after grafts and wound care. PHOTOGRAPH COURTESY OF KELLY STEFFENSEN.

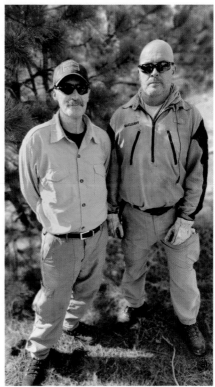

Dan Steffensen and Sean McCleary promoting Yellowstone County Fundraising for Personal Protective Equipment in 2022. PHOTOGRAPH COURTESY OF MIKEL WOLF.

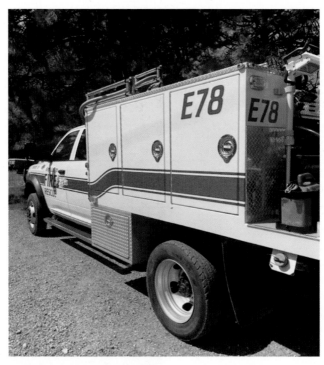

The new E78 Dan took to fight fires in western Montana in August 2023. Mentos in the glove box. PHOTOGRAPH CREDIT DAN STEFFENSEN.

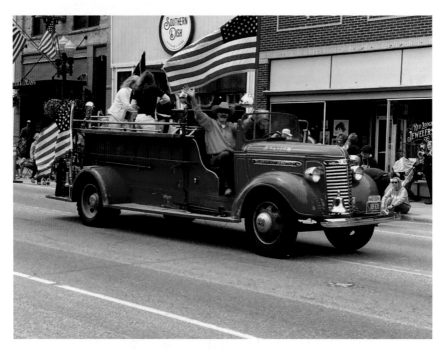

Red Lodge, Montana, on July 4, 2023. Dan was Grand Marshal of the parade. PHOTOGRAPH COURTESY OF CLARK THROSSELL.

Despite the damage and being bound by gauze, Dan was determined to learn how to wipe his ass by himself, which was much harder than it sounds. He says, "They took the catheter out to let me pee on my own; then they had to put it back in. Later, they would do it again, and the nurse said you have to pee by two o'clock, or it goes in again. That's a bigger challenge when they won't let you drink water or even a few ice cubes. It was three o'clock before I did it, and it was all I could do to get the delay and to pee. Putting that in feels like a bowling ball going into your urethra."

He could not swallow correctly. The intubation and the ventilator had damaged the flap needed to avoid aspiration. Dan failed two swallow tests and said he cried like a baby both times. He says, "The feeding tube sucks. It's a teaching hospital, so they asked me if a student could do it. I said yes, and that was an hour of torture."

Dan remembers, "The ice cube was a great game for Kelly, the kids, and me. Sneaking me ice. It was the only pleasure I had."

Dan struggled to believe that life would get any better or that he would be able to function on his own. Kristen Quinn, Utah Medical Psychosocial Program Coordinator and Clinical Mental Health Therapist (CMHC), says, "We must care for the person; then everything falls in line. Knowing there is a life to live helps you have the best chance in that space where you are functional."

The first part of acceptance is acknowledging that there will be a quality of life adjustment. Dan couldn't think of being a firefighter again, and that was unfathomable for him. One of the people who would not let him give up was Erik, who looked for Dan on the floor whenever he was there.

He always approached Dan with, "Get a smile on your face. Let's pull out all the stops. Don't think about how sucky the situation is."

Erik would do everything he could to get Dan through these days. He had seen fire in Dan. But after everything, Dan was still intubated. "I was very concerned after talking to this really cool guy," Erik says. "We all poured our hearts into getting through the first forty-eight hours and ensuring he lived. Statistically, he should not have lived. He can be doing great and, in a flash, go septic and die. Suppose he had known the truth about the months or even one year. Dan would have rolled over and died. He would have lost hope if he knew how completely dependent he was going to be, the next year would be excruciating pain, and he might not recover. There is no promise for a good recovery—sheer hopelessness. You have lost everything."

One day, Dan couldn't wait to tell Erik, "I got to wipe my ass."

Erik said, "Okay then, we've got to get you ready for the Pack Test." The firefighter's test of carrying a forty-five-pound pack for three miles in forty-five minutes seemed impossible to Dan.

Dan said, "I don't know if I can." He had been so proud of finally moving his arm enough to reach his hand around his body, and now Erik was putting another goal in front of him.

Erik said, "There are moderate or minimal Pack Tests."

Dan looked at him with his head down and eyes peering out from under his brow. Erik found Dan jobs that focused on structure protection. For a structure protection specialist, the physical requirements are moderate. Dan could do that job. He was already certified for structures.

Erik said, "You like structures. The physical requirements are moderate."

Still, it was more talk. Dan needed to see it.

Dan would see it in Mark Haley, a Survivor Offering Assistance in Recovery (SOAR, a Phoenix Society[1] program in collaboration with burn centers) Peer Support Volunteer. Mark lost his fingers when badly burned in a race car accident in 2018. He was the first survivor to meet Dan and tell him, "It will get better." At first, Dan didn't want to meet Mark because it meant accepting that he was hurt.

Even though Mark's passion is still antique race cars, he explains that acceptance is the first step to normalcy. After accepting that he was no longer good in the shop, Mark says, "What I can't do was hard to accept. *What can I do* took over my thoughts. My attitude has always been the same as my blood type: B Positive."

Mark spent a year after he left the hospital practicing with the prosthetics when he realized he could drive. There was a big need for drivers. His first job was delivering pharmacy medications. Now, he delivers parts to auto shops.

Dan says, "Mark came to talk to me with lost fingers and an affected foot. I didn't want to talk to another survivor. I was unwilling to accept that I wouldn't have my life back. But I enjoyed talking to him. It was so hard to make my hands start working again. This guy had no fingers. Mark's burns on his legs left him a sliver of muscle, but he walked. *If he can do it, I can do it.* They can tell me all day, but until you see it, you don't believe it."

Dan had prayed to God to stop the pain. He had often imagined and even dreamed about what could have happened if he had fallen down in that field instead of being able to run. He knew he would have never survived lying in a field of flames. Cremation would have come quickly. Everything would have been much better. He says, "If I had died—no pain. No sorrow. Except for the pain and sorrow of my loved ones. And that's what got me out of that fire. I talked to myself all the way through it. No one, even Scott, will ever be able to know or even imagine what that fire was like as it hit me. It was full-on from-the-depths-of-Hell fire. A killer fire that you don't walk away from. But I did."

Now, he wondered if maybe God had been in that field, too. He thought that if the burning bush was the voice of God, then maybe that burning field was Dan's burning bush. God yelled at him then to run, and he was yelling at him now to move.

Did God also send him Mark? If Dan could accept a man like Mark, could he also accept a higher power outside himself?

Erik says, "Dan now dared to ask the question. Two different fitness tests showed that he could still be a firefighter. Okay, there is a way back in to serve his community. He didn't want to hang up his gear. He was proud of his locker."

Erik saw Dan walking more and more and said, "Anytime I saw him, he was walking the unit; he walked with a purpose."

Instead of therapists having to harass Dan to work harder, Dan took the lead. He charged ahead. "Where is PT? We got to get to work. Let's go to wound care. I need to heal."

Meeting Mark, a burn survivor with acceptance and purpose, Dan thought for the first time, "I'm going to recover. I'm going to make that nineteen-lap mile. I'm going to get better."

Dan raised his head high. He said, "Okay, God, we got this."

CHAPTER FOURTEEN

"I want to go home."

Now, EVERYTHING WAS ABOUT GOING HOME.

Tim recalls that Dan was physically in the worst place in the world and was doing everything possible to get discharged. There was so much pain and time involved with the skin grafts without knowing if they worked. "It is terrible how much it takes to get someone through this," Tim says.

When he woke from the coma, one of Dan's first questions was, "Am I going to have to pay for all this shit?" Tim spent many days in Utah and wanted to ensure Dan understood that he wouldn't have to pay for it. His focus had to be on getting better, not worrying about finances. Montana's workers' compensation covered everything, and according to Tim, became the most significant workers' compensation expense in the state's history.

Dan kept telling Tim, "They aren't telling me anything." His tough old bastard syndrome had gotten him through the surgeries and wound care, but his stubborn old fool syndrome was driving his recovery: they always told him things, but he couldn't hear or remember.

The doctor gave Dan a good update in front of Tim and told him he would be there for another couple of months.

Dan admits that he had bitched about the doctors, and he agreed with the "worst patient" label. "Learning to ask for help was hard for me." He was impatient with the people helping him and worked behind their backs to try to heal himself.

Dan hated anything like a bandage or a splint. He removed braces whenever he could so that he could keep moving. This actually helped him heal faster. He exercised his throat, to help him swallow, as well as his hands every morning before the nurses came in. For at least an hour every morning, he exercised and stretched his joints to avoid splints and the possibility of more surgery.

Everywhere in the hospital, there were rules. Dan hates rules. He was and is stubborn about any rule that doesn't make sense to him. "The questions were hard for me for a long time. My name, the date and day, where I was, why I was there. I was always terrified I would answer incorrectly and never be released." But he could see and read the date and time on the whiteboard on the wall across from his bed and realized he could always answer that question when they asked just by reading the wall.

Dan's list of discharge requirements was long. Every member of his family took turns to help him practice, exercise, and walk the required circles around the floor.

They knew he wanted to go home. And they noticed a change in him. He showed his appreciation for their support. It was a nice change from his prior skeptical attitude. For him, the words "I love you" were platitudes. It was just like the word "acceptance." Show me, don't tell me. Dan says, "My values before were, 'This is who I am. I can walk away. Or they can.'" He had been addicted to self-focus, almost like a disease. Now he was appreciative and loving, as if he was being cured.

In Utah, everyone showed Dan how much loving and caring was possible for him. He says, "I was happy to have everyone caring about me. But I reached a point where I knew they had lives to live. I told them I was a big boy. I'll be fine. All I do is lay here, go to PT, go to wound care, and walk when they let me. The bullshit never ended."

Dan wanted to be on his own, alone, again.

The swallow test was his biggest challenge. He couldn't leave until he could swallow and eat on his own. The exercise was noisy, like burping. The speech therapist, Michelle, came in daily to help him, although it wasn't a job requirement. When he recalled how much she helped him, he cried.

Back home, Sarah Ewald was keeping track of the community support and Dan's progress. One day, as she scrolled through social media, a photo became a defining moment. Dan posted a picture that showed off his new ears. He was standing, proud of how far he had come, how hard he had worked just to be able to stand. Sarah Ewald crumbled. The picture tore her in half. She was seeing a robust man who had deteriorated beyond what she ever thought was possible.

Dan had always reminded her of her father. He was her person, her brother, now depleted but with a look of such determination in his eyes. He was focused on recovering. Her knees buckled. Sarah fell to the floor crying.

She ran into Tom's office. "I'm going. I have to see him," she said.

Tom said, "Of course. Go."

Katy joined Sarah on their trip to see Dan for the first time since he was burned. They were a bundle of raw nerves when they walked into the Utah Burn Center. Sarah wanted to encourage him but knew he wouldn't tolerate shallow compliments. She wasn't going to sugarcoat his condition, but she was determined to be strong for him.

The two women entered his room, pausing beside the open heavy wooden doors, waiting for him to realize they were there. Their good friend was tightly wrapped, asleep, almost meager, with his eyes closed, his new ears shiny in the light. The energy in the room was the same as that of a movie theater: walking in quietly, finding a seat, and waiting for the movie to start. Sarah put her hand on Katy's back to steady herself.

"Dan," Sarah almost whispered.

He opened his eyes to make sure he wasn't dreaming. He turned his head towards the almost spiritual sound of his name, and his eyes opened in wide cheer. The man that they loved, Dan, was still there. They rushed to the bed, pulled back at the last moment, and reached out to touch him to make sure he was real.

As quickly as he could, he sat up and lifted his legs to the side of the bed. Dan tried to be tough, but tears streamed down his face. Katy and Sarah were the two women in the firehouse whom he considered sisters or daughters.

"Lordy, have I missed you two," he bawled. They each carefully took one of his gloved hands and cried along.

"You have no idea how much we have missed you," said Sarah.

"I can't hug you guys." He could barely touch them through his bandages. The lack of human touch for the last several weeks caused him physical pain different from the burns and wounds. It created an emptiness. It was an ache for affection.

"We'll be hugging soon enough. You look great," said Katy.

"Yeah, I just had a million-dollar face peel," he said, sniffing and trying to smile.

"I see your humor is still intact," said Katy. The women smiled through their tears.

"What do you think of my new ears?" he asked.

Trying to match his humor, Katy asked, "Can you hear better now?"

Dan's room had turned from dark and quiet as a movie theater to feeling like sunshine, balloons, and ice cream all at the same time. They were excited to show treasures from home. Katy's elementary students had written get-well letters to their hero firefighter. Dan took his time, reading every single letter, cherishing each one. But one grabbed him and threatened to bring back the tears. It was from Ryan Ples's daughter, Chloe.

"She spent thirty minutes thinking about the words," Katy said softly. "She is so meticulous and artistic."

As they continued to read the letters, Dan looked up to see a young boy walk by his room.

"Oh, you have to meet Kevin," he said excitedly. "Kevin! Kevin! Get back here." When the shy boy peeked around the corner, they welcomed him in. The women noticed such an uplifting expression in Dan.

He was giddy while introducing Kevin. The women spent another hour talking to Kevin and showing Dan the letters. When it was time to go, their hearts were lighter. They could see that their friend wanted to come home. He was adamant. He was ready.

Sarah and Kelly met over coffee and started a list of things to do to help Dan come home. At the top of the list was transportation. It had to be by plane. Tom asked Bill Morean in Red Lodge for the use of his private plane. Ruth would have Community Care Service at the ready. There was plenty to do, but they thought it was weeks away when Sarah returned to Red Lodge.

One Zoom meeting later, doctors and family considered the options. Medically, he was good. He passed the tests in the hospital. How many laps could he keep walking around the unit? Though it would be daunting, Kelly could help him with the rest of the wound care at home. The community could care for him at home. There was transport. There was no reason for him to stay in Utah. At the end of the call, Dr. Lewis said that Dan would be leaving in four days.

It all happened so fast. Mandy says, "It was a shock."

Dan was ecstatic. "I'll be fine. This is a battle I have to fight on my own, in my house." So they finally acquiesced to it; Dan was finally going home. Home, where he could feel closer to Marney and have all his things at his fingertips. Home, where he could fight and heal on his own terms. And home, to a town that needed him as much as he needed them.

CHAPTER FIFTEEN

Hero Dan

CHEERING MEN AND WOMEN IN GREEN, PURPLE, AND BLUE SCRUBS lined the hall that circled the floor of the University of Utah Burn Unit. All Dan could hear was the honks of noise makers, whoops, and hollering. The lights and hoops made it seem more like a disco dance floor than a medical facility. Nurses, PTs, doctors, patients, firefighters, and their families all gathered to celebrate the discharge of the burned firefighter.

Dan's release date was shared all over the wildland firefighting community. Emily came in on her day off, and the entire Utah team created a Tunnel of Love to say goodbye. Dan had gone to Kevin's tunnel for an overwhelmingly emotional goodbye. Now, in his own, he held his arms wide to touch hands with everyone.

Emily was so proud of her patient as she watched the sendoff. She says, "Every day, there is a win. Some days, there won't be any progress with someone, and I go home frustrated."

But Dan was going home after just two months, which made sense to people like Danny. "I'm not surprised because he cannot sit still.

Laying there was killing him spiritually. For his sanity, he needed to get out. He had been mummified."

The town of Red Lodge was sending daily outpourings of love. Sarah says, "Our community became a world community overnight. A volunteer wildland firefighter being burned is gripping. We're small. We're Montana." There were boxes of T-shirts on his porch from every fire department in the county—even the world. She counted 385 T-shirts from as far away as Nova Scotia. She also managed the monetary fund that grew into six figures. People would visit Red Lodge and say, "Here is $500 for Dan." They could not keep up with the mail, but Sarah eventually sent a thank you note to everyone.

Dan was just beginning to find out how many people cared about him. Sarah texted Dan and called often. "It was important to hear his voice. I was so unprepared for his resilience and his strength."

When she and Katy visited, they thought they had weeks to prepare for his return. Now, they just had a few days. All hands were now focused on a homecoming. "I told Dan he needed to be prepared for a fanfare," Sarah says. She thought it would help him heal.

A woman visiting Yellowstone heard about the homecoming and came explicitly to welcome him home. She gave the fire station a check because she wanted to be a part of such a momentous occasion. Sarah says, "We just couldn't stop it. The foundation, the paper, the radio. Every Carbon County station and beyond brought a fire engine. We had to control traffic, and all the people wore red."

On September 21, with Tom and a pilot, Dan and Kelly taxied the private airplane onto the Red Lodge runway to love times a thousand. Ambulances, tenders, engines, and their crews from every surrounding town and county created a nest of red, yellow, green, and white colors in celebration of first responders, lined up to welcome home the man considered a miracle. A wildland firefighter miracle.

Dan stepped out of the plane, still covered in protected wraps and proudly wearing a Red Lodge Fire Rescue shirt and hat. He looked around at the crowd with a smile and threw his arms out wide to inhale his hometown.

Dan was overwhelmed. He hugged everyone around the circle, appreciating the physical and emotional connection. "They don't give hugs in the hospital, and I had been hug-deprived and needed every one," he says.

He stopped, stunned, when he realized Sean McCleary and his wife, Kari, stood before him. Sean's brain surgery for his cancer had happened just over two weeks before, and he had been released that morning. The scar was still bright red on the side of his bald head, shiny in the sun. He showed it off proudly to the burned firefighter, who threw his arms around him.

Dan said, "What are you doing here?"

"This is where I need to be," said Sean.

Kari smiled as she explained. "He told me, 'I gotta get out of here, and I'm going to be there to meet Dan.' He insisted."

Dan blubbered. Sean was the other local survivor. They were now brothers fighting a battle of pain and healing and all that goes with it—hospitals, doctors, drugs, insurance, and GoFundMe requests.

The connection between Sean and Dan was more than that of firefighter brothers. They were "Why are we at the center of attention?" brothers, "Everyone thinks we're heroes" brothers, and "No one understands this shit like we do" brothers.

Both men had faced death and survived. Both men were now thinking deeply about their purpose in life. Both men wanted back on a firetruck. *If not that, then what? Who am I if I'm not a firefighter?* Both men said, "If I'm not on a truck, I'm not in the station."

Will understood that kind of thinking as he waited with a huge hug. "They released him early because he was mean," he says. "Erik had said that Dan's attitude depended on how he acted from the beginning. He was looking for that toughness because he was fighting a battle. That competitive thing with Dan resurfaced."

Will adds, "Dan had this horrible *oh shit* moment, and the only thing that separated him from everyone was two steps. This is a story of the perseverance of a good man. He acknowledges the support of his friends and family and has come back with the ability to tackle many things thrown at him in life and come out on the right end. This feeling of him coming home was that we had just achieved a major milestone, a sense of relief and happiness. We all got through this together. Another family member was coming home."

Katy, Tim, and Tom all reached out to welcome Dan. Tim was skeptical at first, but glad Dan was home. The community could now be more proactive in his recovery instead of just worrying about him. Staying in Utah was not in Dan's best interest, and he wasn't the only one that got a little crazy. He had been at the center of Red Lodge's thoughts for so long, and everyone needed him back. It was a huge community relief to have Dan back home, and seeing him smiling and joking lifted everyone's spirits.

Mike Kordenbrock, writing for the *Billings Gazette*, captured the excitement for the hero's return. Katy's fourth grade students were making posters and screaming Dan's name all morning. Jack Exley, Dan's next-door neighbor, had been watching Dan's home and keeping the firefighter's fridge stocked with Dan's favorites: Twinkies and chocolate donuts.[1]

Dan struggled to speak to the crowd waiting to welcome him home—partly because he had never been good at expressing his emotions, but also because of the weeks that he had been lying and then walking with tubes damaging his throat. Still, he found the strength and the words, and then didn't miss giving everyone the long-awaited hug.

Sarah was the last in line—the last hug. Sarah's arms were his first sense of normalcy. Her SUV was waiting to take them to Dan's house, where he would continue his recovery. His only request was to drive through town, not the shortest way across Airport Road. He rolled the windows down just to breathe the essence of the valley. He smiled as they passed Red Lodge Pizza Co., impatient at the thought of ordering one of their pepperoni pizzas. He laughed as they passed Wild Table, owned by Dan's friend Sheena Ernst, anxious to get back to her biscuits and gravy.

As they passed Red Lodge Rescue Fire Station to turn up the hill towards his house, Dan grabbed Sarah's hand and squeezed it tight. Sarah cried with him as they pulled into his neighborhood. The neighbors, including Cathie Osman, waved signs and flags in his driveway.

The entire community was there, jumping, waving, and crying. Cathie says, "We saw the plane circle above our houses for the landing at the airport and waited in his yard, waving flags." She was proud to watch him get out of the car and walk the last 200 feet. The neighbors were confident Dan would be okay in his house with Kelly to help. Plus, Cathie was a physician assistant and her husband Jack Exley was a doctor. The hero firefighter would never have a lack of support.

"The sun was out, and it was a gorgeous day," says Cathie. "Kelly was totally in charge. We mainly listened to see if they needed anything."

Even though everyone else felt good about Dan coming home, it was a huge step. Kelly said the continued care was overwhelming when they returned to Red Lodge. At first, he was a little concerned. Dan's old Red Lodge Fire Rescue shirt swallowed him because it was now five sizes too large. Seeing that, Kelly wondered, "What have we done?"

But the Red Lodge Rescue staff and firefighters were ready to see Dan's recovery through. They took him to doctors' appointments and brought him food. Jon says, "Just knowing he was around was great. The hardest thing for a first responder is being unable to do anything. It's tough when someone is part of your team, and you can't do anything."

Once Kelly understood how much the community needed Dan back home, it helped him realize how important his job was to help Dan recover at home. Kelly was grateful for the support from everyone who came to the house with food, transported the patient to the doctor, and helped with cleaning and bandaging.

Kelly realized being there to care for Dan was the reason his brother could come home early, but his care wasn't just helping Dan. It was helping the town as well. Kelly's time and dedication were a noble act, adding to many others he had given to friends and family.

At times, Kelly needed to be reassured. Cathie Osmun clearly saw the sacrifice. "It was all about Dan. Kelly took all of Dan's anger, all of his irritation, well," she says. "Dan was not at his best. He was in pain. Kelly took all of it for the neighbors."

Kelly had taken on a life-altering job. His brother's daily trauma was something only he could bear to witness. Dan had been a strong man. A tough man. He had lost fifty pounds. Taking a shower required no less than two people standing with him at one time, unwrapping his body of gauze from his neck to his ankles. This was the ritual to begin the horrible indignity of debriding. The pain was barely tolerable on the outside. It was insufferable on the inside.

Just getting up in the morning was an intimidating experience. Dan had to do as much of it himself as possible, so he understood the reality of it. Just as he leaned on the shower wall and his brother, accepting his physical limitations, he also leaned on a higher power. How else could he get through it?

"To us, Dan was gracious," says Cathie. "Caring for him gave us all a chance to be our best selves. Even if it was just to prepare his favorite recipe."

She and Dan began taking long walks to help him prepare for the Pack Test. Besides being a retired Red Lodge Fire Rescue EMT, Cathie is also a breast cancer survivor.

Dan moved in next door to Cathie after Marney died. Her insight into human suffering was inherent because of her experience with chemotherapy. And because of her non-threatening nature, she was the perfect pal for Dan. She describes herself as short and round-faced and says everyone wants to pat her on the cheek.

"Everyone calls me honey or sweetie." Her husband, Jack, is a doctor who, at eighty years old, is now considered Red Lodge Fire Rescue advisory emeritus, meaning he doesn't have to retake the Pack Test.

Cathie and Dan were part of a neighborhood that gathered regularly. "We always had a barbecue once a month, and one was scheduled Friday when Dan was burned," she says. "Dan was bringing a six-pack. When everyone heard a firefighter was hurt in Joliet, the only thought was, 'Who was bringing the beer?' There was no thought that it could be bad or that it was anyone they knew. The news took our breath away. It was a gift that he came home to everyone."

Cathie and Jack were a constant source of encouragement for Dan and Kelly and helped them feel safe. Dan went from 160 pounds to 220 because of his neighbor's mouth-watering recipes. "He likes his carbs," she says. "One day, he told me, 'I think I need to do this myself.'"

Walking with him and talking with him, Cathie got to know her neighbor even better. "Dan is the first one to admit that he is critical, a perfectionist; he wants the system to be perfect to control his world. On the outside, Dan is a gentleman, appreciative, and gracious. Inside, he bitches about everything."

That is who Kelly cared for, with complete understanding and empathy. Kelly knew Dan had reached a point where he wanted everyone gone. But so much of the healing he could not do by himself, especially the compression bandages, which, if applied wrong, would rip the newly grafted skin off. The task of cleaning, bandaging, and moisturizing every inch of his body Dan would have to continue by himself. Kelly had to stay until the firefighter could reach every place he needed to heal.

His kids visited for moral support, but there came a time when they, too, were asked to leave. Margot says, "He appreciated us being there. But then it was time for us to go."

Mandy also understood the request. "He's a doll. We just want him to be a happy doll. It's his choice."

Norman Maclean wrote in *Young Men and Fire*: "His was a story of a tragedy, but tragedy is only a part of it—as it is of life." Dan's story is of surviving, but surviving is only a part of it—as it is of life.

Dan lived but still had to accept his life.

CHAPTER SIXTEEN

"It does get better."

"Between the past and the future is acceptance."[1]

Dan worked very hard to accept his physical appearance and the daily maintenance of his scars. Emotionally, Marney is still everywhere. The table across from the kitchen in Dan's house holds three framed photos of just her. In the living room is a sidebar with more photos lined up. The needlepoint pillows are still against the arms of the couch and every other place to sit. At Christmas, the tree is adorned with her needlepoint ornaments and the fireplace is hung with her needlepoint stockings. Dan still lives emotionally in his past.

Struggling to move on, Dan messaged Mike Maltaverne, "Boy, this thing will not go away."

Mike explains the conflict of a firefighting hero. "It's now part of who he is. Dan is wearing it like armor. The heavy thing he has on him has not seen the level of emotion I know has to be there. We are creating this narrative that he is a tough, strong guy. When does he let out that this sucks? He has a defense mechanism from an immense trauma that won't allow him to go there. This thing is very much alive for him. He gets standing ovations. What a conflict must be going on inside him. The conflict of being put on a pedestal when internally you think you have failed and you think you are fake. He must be saying to himself, 'I'm not who they think I am.'"

Who is he? Since the summer of 2021, Dan has gone from Grumpy Old Man to Tough Old Bastard to Stubborn Old Fool. Each syndrome is a struggle but was needed at the time to keep him going.

Dan read a line from Ernest Hemingway:

"The best people possess a feeling for beauty, the courage to take risks, the discipline to tell the truth, the capacity for sacrifice. Ironically, their virtues make them vulnerable; they are often wounded, sometimes destroyed."

Dan sees this quote as referring to having the courage to be physically wounded or destroyed because that is what he dealt with and survived. "I took this one to heart a long time ago. I think it means to protect and serve each other and the greater community," he says.

But he struggles to understand the vulnerability and the courage needed to be destroyed by emotional wounds. He focuses on physical healing but ignores the courage to connect to the people in his life. These wounds take longer to heal and are thus a greater risk.

It was a year before Dan started having nightmares. At first, he couldn't even admit that he was having them. They were not a consequence of PTSD, but rather a form of Acute Stress Disorder, which is to be expected. He would see flames hitting his face. Or he would dream that he was running from fire.

"These types of dreams usually mean there is something they need to control. You start by focusing on what you can control," says Kristen, who explains the process as Post-Traumatic Growth. At first, it is not unusual for someone like Dan to question if he is glad to be alive. Kristen says, "This is really hard. Often, the only reason to keep fighting is not to see your family suffer."

The main coping skill is mental. It takes time to think and rediscover your values on a deeper level. What seemed important in the past is not important anymore. What could Dan's values become if he was not a firefighter?

Dan finally joined Kristen's survivor support group at the Utah University Burn Center, which helped him and other survivors look deep inside themselves. According to Kristen, the groups are usually men, even though men are generally not group people and don't usually want help. Dan is typical and fits right in.

Kristen says, "In his core self, he likes helping people. Before his burns, he would fix a fence. Now, he has found the space to talk to survivors. When he shares his own feelings, he is helping himself and others at the same time."

Dan compares the mental shift to a chronic illness. "It's taking baby steps. Sitting on the edge of the bed was a big deal. Standing up was a big deal. Each step gets me closer to acceptance and my future. The mental shift is part of getting into the burn community. Burning is forever. Wound care is every freaking day. You think of it as an illness. Like alcoholism is an illness."

This type of illness needs constant therapy, recovery, and group support. The burn group therapy almost parallels alcoholic support. Each step in recovery is closer to acceptance. "I think I'm more accepting," Dan says. "Before, I was not a dick, but I could pull him out when I needed him, like a gun. I could see the dick inside of me close to the surface."

Dan had first started the horribly painful wound care and called back home to Dr. Fouts to tell him he didn't want to live. Dr. Fouts told him he needed to get better because he inspired the town. But that's not what Dan wanted to hear.

Dan says, "That pissed me off. I didn't care about the town. I was worried about me."

As late as February of 2023, Dan was relying on his coping skills of anger and resentment. Even though the doctors told him it would take three years, not even two years in he was impatient. "This piece of shit nightmare that I am in right now, healing is not what I am used to."

Dan turned some of his control over to a higher power but was not quite connecting all the dots. He accepted he could recover when he saw Mark and talked with Erik, which motivated him. But he didn't feel like a firefighter anymore. That non-feeling would be there for the next two years. His future was still in doubt.

"Two years down the fucking road, I'm still trying to heal. The loss of being a firefighter is all I had to replace Marney. And now that is being threatened. I recognize that and truly wonder how I can get past that loss. I'm dead inside."

When he was an alcoholic, he was restless, irritable, and discontented. At one time, he used whiskey or beer to drown his sadness, but Dan no longer copes with drinking. Still, being burned screwed with his identity so much that he was forced to take inventory of his life. Like a step in recovering from alcoholism, he was coming to terms with who he was before and who he wanted to become.

Norman Maclean wrote about smokejumpers in *Young Men and Fire*: "The 'it' is within, and is the need to settle some things with the universe. It's something special within that demands we do something special."

Dan did something special. It should have killed him.

But he lived to face the high stakes of being a burn survivor. According to his fellow survivor and now brother Mark, the high stakes is a return to normalcy, which for Mark is fatherhood; the ability to function was secondary.

Mark says, "People compliment me on my ability to use my hooks, which annoys me because I'm just getting my wallet out of my pocket. I want normalcy. There is a past and a future, and where they meet is acceptance."

Is Dan's return to normalcy being driven by ego, a self-seeker taking risks to maintain his character? He said normalcy for him was to get back to where he was. Is that the highest he can set the bar? If the higher power is in control, couldn't he go even higher? He says, "I started to accept it when I met Mark. I counted all my fingers, and I knew how lucky I was."

Accepting his physical reality is only a part of it. "My lips will never be right. Mandy said, 'Put that cream on them. They look awful.' You should see them from this side." Some things may never be normal, but the ability to function is secondary.

Does he want to return to the same mental and emotional normalcy? Dan admits to being ego-centric, taking high risks, and being obsessive-compulsive. He keeps his house as clean as he sweeps the floor of the firehouse garage. These are all traits consistent with an addictive personality. Other traits include being disconnected from people and wanting to control your environment.

Dan's environment blew up. He was swathed for weeks with no control of his hands and bodily functions. He could not manage scratching his nose, let alone controlling his life, and was forced to seek help, similar to what an alcoholic has to accept. At that moment, in tremendous pain and needing to put everything he had into recovery, it was impossible for Dan to think of anyone but himself. He could not heal himself. He could not move. The darkness in his room pierced inside his soul and the broken part of his mind.

Maybe because of his Mormon childhood, maybe because he had recovered from alcoholism, Dan leaned on a higher power to find a light. Dan had long talks with God in Utah. He prayed for himself in

Utah, and when he returned to Red Lodge, he still prayed about himself. "God saved *me* for a reason." He is still ego-driven.

It has not been easy for him to think outside of himself. The world idolizes him as a hero and an inspiration. It is impossible not to have an ego living with such admiration. But did he himself, by himself, get through the suffering and the hurt?

No, and he knows it. He prayed to God. And just possibly, God answered by sending him a thousand angels in the form of rescue, medicine, honor guards, therapy, workers' comp, friends, and family.

Dan keeps asking, "What does God want me to do?" The answer may be nothing. Maybe the answer is simply to love others like himself—his fellow burn survivors. He relates to them because of their similar struggles: the injuries, the uncertainty, the nightmares, the pain, and a new life of forever maintenance. They are his new brothers, just like firefighter brothers. With them, he knows who he is and how to be. They are like him and don't challenge him to connect beyond the complex subjects of burns and firefighting. With them, he can step outside himself and maybe raise the bar.

But what about his blood family or friends? He says, "My values have changed so that I am open to deeper personal relationships, but I'm particular."

Layne considers Existential Therapy helpful for first responders. The therapy focuses on "givens."[2] One given is that humans have the freedom and responsibility to create meaningful lives. The other givens are that humans are ultimately alone, life can feel meaningless, and death is inescapable. An alcoholic would follow these "givens" with the belief that you find meaning only through a higher power.

Does Dan feel a responsibility to find a meaningful life? He has spent the last two years unable to feel like a firefighter, a lifestyle that had fed his ego, giving him meaning. Is returning to where he was enough to create a meaningful life? Does ego get in the way of giving up control to a higher power? Isn't egoism an isolating and lonely pursuit?

Dan maintains relationships through texting and keeping people in his phone more than in his life. Connecting with Dan on a deeply personal level is usually one-sided. Without him knowing it, his lack of energy towards or prioritizing people makes his friends or family feel he pushes them away.

His least egoic and most loving attitudes are with his burn brothers and sisters. In this world, he has experienced who he is with and without God. He has lived a horrible life and knows that God saved him. Only divine intervention could have given him the instant forethought not to breathe when the fire aimed for his throat and lungs.

He says, "I was closer to God for months. We discussed things. We discussed whether or not I wanted to live. I always had the choice to die. I should have died, Sean should never have had cancer, and Ryan should never have died. I want to know what God wants me to do with the rest of my life."

Dan keeps asking the question. Maybe the answer is not outside of him, but inside. It's not what he can do. It's what he can become. Could he become in his heart and mind a walking testimonial, a message of love and grace? No one can do or give any more than that.

"Love your neighbor as yourself" seems as much a cure as a commandment. Is it possible to achieve that high of a bar? Is that what Dan can become—a man full of love for others? Can he become a person able to love deeply and wholly? Or is the question: How much can he love himself?

Dan says opening himself up to tell his story has been like Cartman in *South Park* being probed by aliens. "I have to face the fact that feeding my ego got me into this. Not this fire, not this day. But my desire to be the best firefighter I could be. I think ego is what makes us put out fires and win wars."

Dan read a novel called *Dear Edward* about a kid who survived a plane crash that killed 191 people, including his brother and parents. He received hundreds of letters, many from the families of others killed in the crash. Most of them said he was spared for a reason and needed to do what they suggested to fulfill that gift. The character in the book goes to a tarot card reader who is a reincarnation of one of the passengers on the plane. And she tells him, "There was no reason for what happened to you. It was dumb luck. Nobody chose you for anything."

When he read that in the book, Dan couldn't make sense of anything anymore. He was in a horrific plane crash when he was eighteen and walked away mostly unhurt, although the others were hurt pretty badly. People then told him he was saved for a reason.

Now again, he wonders, "What the fuck is the reason? So I can live through heartache, pain, sorrow, losing Marney, and killing her under the guise of hospice? The sadness outweighed the happiness. And then to be tested yet again by the fire."

The character in the book *Dear Edward* talked about meeting his shrink. Dan says, "He said exactly what I said to Chief Maltaverne. 'I feel I should be over it by now. Everyone else has forgotten about the flight. But I feel like I still think about it all the time. And I do. All day, every day.'"

Edward's shrink answered, "What happened was baked into your bones. It lives under your skin. It's part of you and will be part of you until you die."

Dan thought this was ironic. He tells this writer, "It is baked into my bones. And it will live *on* my skin, not in it. What I've been working on since I first met you is part of learning to live with it. That's what my shrink is, and in many ways, you are, by writing this book for me, helping me deal with that."

Post-Traumatic Growth

As Dan dealt with his emotional and physical scars, the residents of Red Lodge tried to find their own sense of normalcy. Had they accepted what happened that summer? Was Dan coming home enough for them to return to normalcy? No.

Layne says, "It's common not to accept it. Firefighters are supposed to be immune from getting hurt. You think you did something wrong, even when you didn't."

The International Association of Fire Fighters has determined that balanced wellness is essential for all firefighters, so much so that testing beyond Pack Tests is being implemented in firehouses nationwide. Wellness is "intended to strengthen uniformed personnel so that their mental, physical, and emotional capabilities are resilient enough to withstand the stresses and strains of life and the workplace."[3]

Resiliency is coping with stressful events in life, especially if you learn from the event. The Fire Service Joint Labor Management wellness-Fitness Initiative reports that "Acceptance, humor, religion, and positive reframing [are] among the top coping strategies" for firefighters. "They create a sense of meaning and eventually accept the 'new normal' of their lives following a traumatic event."[4] First responders are always dealing with death and suffering. To cope, they must find meaning in suffering or learn how to live by accepting the human suffering of death.[5] Caring and supportive relationships are essential to finding meaning. After that summer, the relationships in Red Lodge are as solid as the granite the town is built upon.

Red Lodge Fire Rescue discovered how deeply they could lean on each other with their undaunted, trusting relationships. Sarah and Ruth; Tyler, Hank and Danny; all the chiefs, Tom and Will; and every firefighter, EMT, and SAR became closer with each other and the townspeople. Amy says, "It was a good thing it was us. We had the relationships and the leadership necessary to get through it. No one ever said we could have done better. The thread running through each pillar supports the other. Search and Rescue had Tate, Fire had Dan, and the town never faltered."

Cathie Osmun adds, "People coming to help amid a nightmare is not quantifiable."

Dan says, "Understanding that you are not alone is a big mental shift. When you realize this is forever, accept it and everything it entails—scars and grafts to maintain, that I may need more help, what my new life looks like—it's easier to cope."

This is a statement from a man who always hated asking for help but who has accepted that his life has changed—that there is a power greater than himself waiting just outside the window, ready to be called upon when the next storm comes. He has experienced that what is beyond his control is best left to God.

The same is true for Red Lodge Fire Rescue and the town. The summer of 2021 was a series of horrible tragedies beyond their control. Their response is to focus on what they can control. They talk to each other, find common causes such as remembering Tate as they train for SAR, memorialize Ryan Ples on the ski slope, and celebrate Dan coming home. To give meaning, they mark every moment of sadness and gladness.

The Utah University Hospital Health Burn Center's staff does the same, celebrating every win with their Tunnel of Love. They, too, need a form of closure and ceremony. Dan's leaving memorialized their work as they sent him off to his new beginning. He was not healed, but he was prepared.

Sarah says, "The town has not healed yet. We each relive the experience in different ways. We don't need to heal. We learned from it to prepare for the next unknown."

The community came together, but the memories are never gone any more than Dan's scars are gone from his skin. There is no pretending that it never happened. There is a knowledge that they are capable of handling hard things. There is growth. You don't know you have grown until something like this happens. Tom knows it and sleeps well at night.

Dan opened one of the big garage fire station doors on Broadway, squinting as he let in the morning sun. He was sure he was dreaming. He could smell coffee brewing from down the street, mixed with the tasty freshness of the mountain air. He turned back into the garage and saw that he wasn't dreaming.

He didn't move, staring at the new E78 parked in the middle of the garage, white and clean, sparkling with life. Dan looked down at the sponge in his hand that he had grabbed to wash the other engines that morning. Then he looked back at E78. He tried to move closer but could only point with the sponge.

"How do you like it?" asked Tom. He had just walked into the station and realized Dan was looking at the new engine. Tom was almost giddy.

"Wait, I want to be with you when you see it," said Sarah as she bound down the stairs and rushed to be by Dan's side. "And don't forget these." She pulled an unwrapped roll of Mentos out of her pocket and showed them to him.

Dan put his free hand around hers with the Mentos in her palm. He clasped it hard and did not let go.

Tyler joined them from his office, beaming. "Okay, Dan, let's get you back in there," he said, slapping Dan on the back to urge him forward.

Dan took the Mentos from Sarah's hand. "I got this."

He took ten steps, opened the passenger door to E78, climbed into the passenger seat, opened the glove box, and put the Mentos inside. He thought he heard the engine whisper to him, "Welcome back, boss."

As a firefighter, Dan only wanted to be the best he could be. He did not seek to be a hero. Surviving, healing, and coming home to Red Lodge,

Montana, a town that needed him to come home, is why he is a hero. The inhuman ordeal of living through the pain and recovery of burns is why Dan is inspirational. Now, he hopes to add value to the burn survivor and firefighter communities. That may be the best way he can love others like himself.

Dan is a firefighter.

In Memoriam
Captain Sean McCleary
Father, Husband, Friend, Firefighter
June 16, 1969–July 13, 2023

Epilogue

In the Spring of 2022, Dan and Sean gave their time to be in a marketing campaign produced by the students of Montana State University Billings to raise money for Personal Protective Equipment for local firefighters.

In the Summer of 2022, Dan was in Utah for more skin grafts when the "500-year rain" resulted in the entire Yellowstone River Shed flooding. Rock Creek overran Red Lodge with no warning. There was tremendous damage to the town and throughout Montana as a result. The northern entrances to the park and many cities were left devastated for most of the summer and into 2023. Once again, this was the community, just as this was the man, to endure disaster. They knew they were prepared, united, and tough enough to survive.

In October of 2022, Dan revisited the burn site of the bluff on Farewell Road for the first time since the burnover. It was a sunny day with a strong breeze. The view of the Beartooth Mountains was clear. He retraced where his engine drove through the cut hole in the fence and where he attacked the fire along the edge of the bluff. He looked to the west to point out how it was impossible to see a thunderstorm because another bluff blocked the view on the horizon. He described where he stood and hugged the side of the engine as the fire blasted under it to find him and then how he ran and jumped over the fence. Dan was calm, reflective, and happy to soak in the panoramic view and inhale the fresh air.

Driving away from the bluff that day, he passed by and saw his friend Larry Vukonich working in front of his new house. Dan stopped his truck, got out, and surprised his good friend with a big hug. Larry says, "I always knew he would be fine; he's tough."

On November 14, 2022, Dan tested his scarred and grafted skin in the training tower and texted, "I did two evolutions in the fire room. I did not feel pain anywhere at about 350 degrees at shoulder height. Pretty excited about that. Would have liked to test the legs more, but I feel good about it."

On May 18, 2023, Dan texted *43:10*. It was his time on the Pack Test, physically qualifying him to fight fires for Red Lodge Fire Rescue.

On May 23, 2023, Dan had one last skin graft on the back of his left leg. Dr. Thompson was giddy to find fresh donor skin on his right thigh to pull as the donor site. Soon after, he could go without wearing any bandages anywhere on his body.

On July 30, 2023, Dan returned to full-time duty at Red Lodge Fire Rescue, two years and fourteen days after being burned.

On August 4–9, 2023, Dan was a counselor at a camp for the burn survivor "littles" in Utah. Kevin was a camper.

On August 19, 2023, Dan took the new E78 to help fight fires in Western Montana.

Encore: "Did I do something wrong?"

When he was burned over, Dan's first reaction to Jeff and Tim was, "I fucked up."

Will says, "First and foremost, you have to look at the actions of his crew member, Scott Wilson. He did exactly what Dan had briefed him to do. Don't panic. Go to the black and stay in the engine. What might have happened if Dan hadn't briefed him? Good job, Dan. Good job, Dan."

Even after he awoke from the coma, Dan questioned, "Did I do something wrong?" His mentor, Tyler, asked himself, "Did I not teach him enough?"

Dan's love of firefighting had always been about solving the puzzle: how to fight it safely, teach the next recruit, recognize a great firefighter, and be the best mentor he could be.

Mike Maltaverne, assistant chief of Bozeman and now chief of Driggs, Idaho, talked about the learning analysis and how the first responders put pressure on themselves. "We were conscious about how we portrayed the people and the events to share the story so people could learn from it. It is an extraordinary story, and we felt compelled to protect the people because the incident emotionally changed them. We were careful about working with respect for Dan and his colleagues."

Bad and sick are not enough to describe how people felt. Mike, who has been a firefighter for thirty-two years, was struck by the fact that he'd been in the same situation as Dan dozens of times. "From the moment he left the station, they checked their equipment, checked the weather, and reviewed their plan. I empathize because I've been in their shoes, but I've been lucky. I never realized how lucky I've been. And then you meet Dan. I get emotional just thinking about him. We are so similar. There have been times when my only purpose was the fire department."

It was like looking in the mirror for Mike. "It could have been me. As soon as the burnover occurred, all Dan was thinking about was everybody else. That day, he was concerned about everyone else, especially his partner. Dan told Scott the day they came together, 'You did a good job. You didn't panic.' Dan was standing there with his body burned. It was okay if he thought about himself, but he couldn't do it. It's changed how I approach the job. It's affected me. I take the job much more seriously. I learned my lesson from Dan. We had to get the analysis right. We told the story as accurately as we could."

Mike says Chief Hoferer was another remarkable man. He had a lot of respect for a man at the sunset of his life, still dedicated to his town, Joliet. "His integrity and loyalty, no one else will do it—volunteer with no resources, high risk, and high liability. He got hit hard with reality. Normally, a job worrying about if there will be enough money next year for car fuel. But this is the ultimate fear of any of us in leadership. It keeps us all awake. In small communities with no resources, everyone was focused on Dan and his condition. But there was still a huge fire burning. Melvin was brushed aside, and no one checked on him. He was about as raw as they come. Two weeks later. We had taken mental health for granted. We learned you have to get resources out there for mental health."

All the reviewers were ICs, and Mike wondered if there was a silver bullet. "There was a briefing. He was monitoring conditions, but Chief Hoferer nailed it. He was a textbook. He had the incident set up well. But they had a weather event. I closed the loop at the fire chief conference in Missoula. Melvin was emotional. I told him, IC to IC, 'You did nothing wrong.' The look on his face was that of a man who had just crawled out of a grave."

Melvin said, "You don't know; I'm not sleeping at night. I need to hear this."

Mike told him, "You had it just how we trained it to be. You just didn't have a crystal ball."

Just before the incident, the NWS in Billings clocked sixty-mile-an-hour gusts thirty miles west in Big Timber. No one on the fire would have received notice. "They were just getting set up. A little three-acre fire north of Joliet was not reported to NWS. Just get on scene, do a size up, look at the conditions, people start arriving, get them set, check resources, call for air support, everything takes time. They had just got on the scene. Remember, Dan was in the first wave. The response to the fire was still occurring when Dan was burned. They were still unpacking the incident. Joliet and Red Lodge engines were effective in knocking the fire down. It was set up well by the chief. The helicopter was overhead. Jeff was on his way. NWS had just picked up the wind event. An hour too late. NWS was typing it up. 'Outflow winds, we should put out an advisory.' Maybe ten minutes later, Jeff would have gotten the info. The timing was terrible."

Mike is a student of the game and is invested in the story because he realizes it could have been him. Then he met Dan and became emotionally involved with him.

The analogy of Dan solving the puzzle fits. Think of the puzzle on a table. The corners and the edges are complete. Then the wind comes up and blows the table over. An IC has all the pieces of the puzzle. There was only so much time to put the pieces together, but the table got bumped, and the IC had to start all over: contingency plans, safety zones, escape routes, plan B, and plan C. In this case, the table blew over before they got the pieces out of the box.

The Joliet engine came over to assist and witnessed Dan and Scott still trying to pump water. Scott shut the pump down. Scott looked for Dan, stumbling around, looking for his helmet, which had blown away and burned up.

Mike concludes, "The real takeaway is Dan's character; this story's human side is that this guy did everything right, but sometimes bad things happen. How awesome how Dan responded. He cared about the firefighter assigned to him. He cared about everybody still left to fight the fire. Instead of himself, he's worried that he screwed up. That's his character."

Melvin couldn't sleep at night until he finally met Mike Maltaverne. Mike told Melvin that from the moment the fire started to the time of the burnover, there was no time to do anything differently. They had just got there. They were just setting up. Everybody did the right thing. The training kicked in. Everyone reacted quickly and got Dan medical assistance right away. It helped that Dan recovered.

"The best day of my life was when he came home," says Melvin. "All hell broke loose. What should I have done? On all our parts, it makes it hard for us to sleep at night for some time. Waist high grass sagebrush within. It was what Hell looks like."

Melvin still gets emotional about it. He felt some guilt because he was the IC and ultimately responsible. "It was my watch. By the time I got on the scene and asked for a spot check. I would not have gotten it back in time. Jeff wasn't there yet." They hadn't set up long enough to even change over radio channels. Melvin had serious doubts about his ability until he read the report. "If I did something wrong, the consequence was a man being burned."

Everyone related to that event felt guilty and questioned if they did something wrong. Even paramedic Marla Frank, who saved Dan's life in the first twenty minutes, questions herself. "Should I have forced pain medicine on him even though he refused? Should I have covered him in moist towels, or would that have given him hyperthermia?"

Danny says, "The four of us, Tyler, Will, Hank, and I, sat up many nights around the fireplace, drinking too much, and threw logs on the fire. Talking about the summer of shit. None of us dealt with it well. We had each other. Too much ego. A lot of self-doubt and criticism. What we should have done, what we did. What we can do going forward. We should have trained harder in ever-changing conditions. The NWS didn't know we were there. Call for spot weather on the way now. We know where we are going. Let them know we are putting people in harm's way. Not given enough information. Let everyone know. You should always ask. There was a communication issue. Missed LCES. Scott was not the most experienced; the most experienced should be your lookout."

Erik says, "I am not surprised by his emotional struggles. Some can't even look at their burns. It represents that 'I messed something up on a test; I should have known better.' It's a permanent mark, especially for firefighters. 'Damn, how often do we train to be aware of the wind or this fuel type? A watch-out situation. How fucking stupid could I have been?' He must be thinking that. Even though the report says, he did nothing wrong, especially with being responsible for Scott. Imposter syndrome is going on."

Danny says, "Some are not equipped to deal with depression. They put the bad stuff in a box. You must open the box, remove the pieces, and go through it like spring cleaning. Or you will explode and be a puddle. We deal with it together."

Tim reflects on the experience: "It could have been me—the consequences have affected all of us. Firefighting was always exciting and thrilling, even working thirty hours at a time. I never thought about it. What we went through with Dan shows us this is difficult and dangerous. I just never thought about it before Dan. The ripple effect on every single person who had a part in his recovery is far-reaching. You just think a bit more and take the shine off of being a firefighter."

Facilitated Learning Analysis (FLA), conducted by the Montana DNRC.

According to Chief Mike Malteverne, an FLA is not an investigation but is a process to maximize opportunities to learn from unintended outcomes or near-miss events, as in this case, the burnover involving Dan. The intent is to share among firefighting professionals and improve performance by generating interest and conversations in a learning environment. The specific details of the incident are not as important as an overall understanding of the event to support discussion.

This process was ordered by Montana Department of Natural Resources and Conservation and assembled subject matter experts from DNRC staff, Montana Fire Wardens, Montana Fire Chiefs and an expert in the FLA process.

A complete Facilitated Learning Analysis, can be found at https://wildfiretoday.com/documents/Harris%20Fire%20Burnover_FLA.pdf.

Bibliography

Buffet, Jimmy. "The Captain and the Kid." Track 1 on Jimmy Buffet, *Down to Earth*. Barnarby Records. 1970.

Burke, Minyvonne. "Body of Montana hiker found under rocks nearly 2 months after she vanished." NBC News. August 24, 2021. www.nbcnews.com/news/us-news/body-montana-hiker-found -under-rocks-nearly-2-months-after-n1277545.

California Department of Forestry and Fire Protection. "Thomas Fire." n.d. www.fire.ca.gov/incidents/2017/12/4/thomas-fire/.

Center for Disease Control and Prevention. "Coronavirus Disease 2019 (COVID-19)." February 11, 2020. www.cdc.gov/ coronavirus/2019-ncov/index.html.

Conlon, Casey. "Laurel Firefighter Paying It Forward After Double Brain Tumor Removal." Q2 News (KTVQ). January 31, 2023. www.ktvq.com/news/positively-montana/laurel-firefighter-pay ing-it-forward-after-double-brain-tumor-removal.

Desmond, Matthew. *On the Fireline: Living and Dying with Wildland Firefighters*. University of Chicago Press. 2007. Quoted in The University of Chicago Press, n.d. www.press.uchicago.edu/Misc/ Chicago/144085.html.

FireScape Mendocino. "August Complex Fire." n.d. www.firescape mendocino.org/august-complex-fire/.

Fox 5 San Diego. "Santa Anna Winds Fuel Growing Thomas Fire." December 14, 2017. www.fox5sandiego.com/news/santa -ana-winds-fuel-growing-thomas-fire/.

Gabbert, Bill. "Report Released for Burnover on the Harris Fire Near Joliet, MT." Wildfire Today. January 19, 2022. www.wildfiretoday .com/2022/01/19/report-released-for-burnover-on-the-harris-fire -near-joliet-mt/.

Goffman, Erving. *Where the Action Is: Three Essays.* Allen Lane The Penguin Press, London, 1969.

Historic Montana. "Red Lodge City Hall and Fire Station: Red Lodge Commercial Historic District." n.d. www.historicmt.org/items/show/142?tour=8&index=19.

International Association of Fire Fighters. "The Fire Service Joint Labor Management Wellness-Fitness Initiative." IAFC.org. www.iafc.org/docs/default-source/1safehealthshs/wfi-manual.pdf.

Kashyap, Neha. "Existential Therapy Techniques and Benefits." Verywell Health. January 24, 2024. www.verywellhealth.com/existential-theory-5272172.

Kordenbrock, Mike. "MT Firefighter Returns Home After Burn Treatments." Firehouse. September 22, 2021. www.firehouse.com/safety-health/news/21239343/mt-firefighter-returns-home-after-burn-treatments.

Kordenbrock, Mike. "Seriously Burned MT Wildland Firefighter Has Second Surgery." Firehouse, July 23, 2021. www.firehouse.com/safety-health/news/21231606/seriously-burned-mt-wildland-firefighter-has-second-surgery.

MacLean, Norman. *Young Men and Fire.* University of Chicago Press. 1992.

Maxouris, Christina. "The largest wildfire in California is finally contained." CNN. September 20, 2018. www.cnn.com/2018/09/20/us/california-mendocino-complex-fire-contained-trnd/index.

MTN News. "Man Who Started Robertson Draw Fire Sentenced to 10 Years in Prison." Q2 News (KTVQ). August 18, 2022. www.ktvq.com/news/crime-watch/man-who-started-robertson-draw-fire-sentenced-to-10-years-in-prison.

National Archives. "Treaty of Fort Laramie (1868)." March 29, 2022. www.archives.gov/milestone-documents/fort-laramie-treaty.

National Center for Health Statistics. "Deaths by Week and State."
Centers for Disease Control and Prevention, n.d. www.cdc.gov/
nchs/nvss/vsrr/COVID19/index.htm.

National Wildfire Coordinating Group. "NWCG Incident Response
Pocket Guide (IRPG)." n.d. www.nwcg.gov/sites/default/files/
publications/pms841.pdf.

The National Institute for Occupational Safety and Health. "FFFIPP –
Data and Statistics." n.d. www.cdc.gov/niosh/fire/data.html.

NBC Montana. "Robertson Draw Fire Just Under 30,000 Acres
Burned, 65% Contained." July 3, 2021. www.nbcmontana.com/
news/local/robertson-draw-fire-just-under-30000-acres-burned
-65-contained.

Q2 News (KTVQ). "Red Lodge Ready for Fourth of July Weekend."
July 2, 2021. www.ktvq.com/news/local-news/red-lodge-ready
-for-fourth-of-july-weekend.

Sage, Jeremy L. and Nickerson, Norma P. "The Montana Expression
2017: 2017's Costly Fire Season." 2017. Institute for Tourism and
Recreation Research Publications. www.scholarworks.umt.edu/
itrr_pubs/363.

University of Utah Health. "Burn Center." January 24, 2024.
www.healthcare.utah.edu/burncenter/.

USAFacts. "Montana Coronavirus Cases and Deaths." February 8,
2024. www.usafacts.org/visualizations/coronavirus-covid-19
-spread-map/state/montana/.

Western Montana History. "Red Lodge Montana." n.d. www.western
mininghistory.com/towns/montana/red-lodge/.

Endnotes

Chapter 1

1 This area was Crow Country for over 400 years. Once coal and gold were discovered, the area started to be settled around 1882. In 1886, the Fort Laramie treaty resettled Crow Country eastward, including the ancient Pryor Mountains, worn down to smooth rumps compared to their immediate neighbor, the towering Beartooth Mountains. Coal mining was the main industry until the 1930s. The historic main street, which is perfect in size for a Western movie set, traces its roots to the early settlers of Montana. Jeremiah Johnson was once the constable. The Beartooth Highway opened in 1930, linking Red Lodge to Yellowstone National Park. National Archives, "The Treaty of Fort Laramie (1868)" & Western Montana History, "Red Lodge Montana."

Chapter 2

1 Kordenbrock, "Seriously Burned MT Wildland Firefighter Has Second Surgery."

2 The Thomas Fire affected Ventura and Santa Barbara Counties, destroying 1,063 structures and over 281,000 acres. CAL Fire, "Thomas Fire."

3 Desmond, *On the Fireline: Living and Dying with Wildland Firefighters.*

Chapter 3

1 Center for Disease Control and Prevention, "Coronavirus Disease 2019 (COVID-19)."

2 Usage of the Emergency Management Assistance Compact (EMAC), where a governor of one state asks the governor of another state for help, peaked in 2017: "Montana, along with many western states, experienced a severe fire season. . . . The NRCC estimates the total costs of fighting Montana's wildfires topped $390 million. . . . The combination of extreme firefighting costs and lower than expected revenues generated a $200 million shortfall with the state government." Sage & Nickerson, "The Montana Expression 2017: 2017's Costly Fire Season."

3 FireScape Mendocino, "August Complex Fire."

4 The lookout is critical to the fight and the plan, often with the most experienced firefighter assigned to the role. After assessing the weather and fire behavior, Order #2 requires firefighters to watch the fire constantly. In the firefighter's Incident Response Pocket Guide (IRPG), four critical tasks must be implemented to ensure firefighter safety: Lookouts, Communications, Escape Routes, and Safety Zones (LCES). The lookout should be an experienced, competent, and trusted firefighter. They must find and maintain a location that provides views of the fire and the crews and good radio communications.

5 The incident commander is responsible for ensuring the system operates properly and the team is as safe as possible. The IC sets the strategy and tactics and assigns the team tasks. Firehouse.com, "Duties & Responsibilities Of The Incident Commander."

6 Goffman, "Where the Action Is."

7 Desmond, *On the Fireline: Living and Dying with Wildland Firefighters.*

8 Heart attacks and strokes are the leading cause of death among firefighters; next are incidents involving vehicles. NWCG, "NWCG Incident Response Pocket Guide."

Chapter 4

1 Originally, the Red Lodge City Fire Department had three paid employees to care for the horses that pulled the water wagon. The rest were volunteers for structure fires in the community. Now Red Lodge Fire Rescue handles wildland and structure and motor vehicle fires, accidents, swift water, backcountry, other rescues, emergency medical calls, and other emergency and non-emergency requests for assistance in Red Lodge and surrounding areas in Carbon County. It has three structure engines, five wildland engines, three water tenders, two rescue vehicles, two incident management vehicles, five ambulances—three in Red Lodge, one in Roberts, and one in Luther—and several ancillary vehicles. Fire, Search and Rescue (SAR), Emergency Medical Services (EMS) make up Red Lodge Fire Rescue.

2 National Wildlife Coordinating Group, "Incident Response Pocket Guide (IRPG)."

3 Black is where the fire has already burned, making it a safe zone or escape route.

4 John Lightburn of Roberts was sentenced to ten years in prison. MTN News, "Man Who Started Robertson Draw Fire Sentenced to 10 Years in Prison."

5 National Wildfire Coordinating Group, "NWCG Incident Response Pocket Guide (IRPG)."

6 Dan didn't have a weather check on that first day when the fire started. When it, or any fire, becomes a Type 1 or 2 fire, an incident meteorologist is usually assigned to the fire.

7 The Community Care organization was born in Red Lodge as a test pilot for the Montana State Health and Human Service Department. The organization takes on all non-emergency referrals from Dr. Fouts, Medical Director of Red Lodge Fire Rescue. All the EMTs operate

under Dr. Fouts' medical license. He is also a local physician to many area residents, including Dan.

8 Q2 News (KTVQ), "Red Lodge Ready for Fourth of July Weekend."

Chapter 5

1 Severity: Assigned to the state to be on call for any fire in the county.

2 Hasty means what it says: a team that moves quickly.

3 At the height of COVID, in the fall of 2020, Carbon County had seventy new cases per day. USAFacts, "Montana Coronavirus Cases and Deaths."

Chapter 6

1 Gabbert, "Report Released for Burnover on the Harris Fire Near Joliet, MT."

Chapter 7

1 The Harris Fire Learning Analysis summarized the incident: "At 16:18 on July 16th, 2021, an ambulance was requested for a burn victim near Joliet, Montana. The call came 58 minutes after the smoke plume was reported for the fire, 40 minutes after the engine carrying the firefighter arrived on the scene, and about 10 minutes after the engine first engaged with the fire."

2 https://healthcare.utah.edu/burncenter/.

3 Prepping him for the flight meant calculating for fluids to make sure his kidneys were working, a sedation plan with the flight crew, good intubation so that his lungs were functioning, and medication for pain if needed. The plan is driven by protocol. Dan had IV lines with automatic pumps and a ventilator to control the protocol throughout the flight. The flight crew printed off his medication list from his primary doctor on the way to Utah.

Chapter 9

1 From the ambulance bay, an injury this severe bypasses the emergency department and goes right to the ICU burn unit. The room is prepared on the front end with enough vacuum and oxygen plugs in the wall to monitor blood pressure, respiration, oxygen intake, and pulse. Dan would use all twelve plugs in the wall.

Chapter 10

1 Maxouris, "The largest wildfire in California is finally contained."

2 Kordenbrock, "Seriously Burned MT Wildland Firefighter Has Second Surgery."

Chapter 11

1 Burke, "Body of Montana hiker found under rocks nearly 2 months after she vanished."

Photo Gallery

Chapter 13

1 www.phoenix-society.org, Phoenix Society for Burn Survivors.

1 The long black tape was diagonally pressed across the side doors on wildland fire engines during California's Thomas Fire in 2017—the sign of a fatality. ABC News reported that "Cory Iverson, 32, of Escondido, California, died while battling the Thomas fire in Ventura and Santa Barbara counties." ABC News, "Firefighter Dies While Battling California Wildfire."

Chapter 15

1 Kordenbrock, "MT Firefighter Returns Home after Burn Treatments."

Chapter 16

1 Credited to Kristen Quinn Burn Group.

2 Kashyap, "Existential Therapy Techniques and Benefits."

3 "Wellness is a term that refers to an individual's state of mind as well as their physical state, balancing between health and physical, mental, emotional and spiritual fitness. . . . Moreover, wellness should be an interactive process where an individual becomes aware of and practices healthy choices to establish a balanced lifestyle." IAFF, "The Fire Service Joint Labor Management Wellness-Fitness Initiative."

4 Ibid.

5 Other therapies that are tools for healing, Layne said, include Cognitive Behavioral Therapy, EMDR or Eye Movement Desensitisation Reprocessing, and Accelerated Resolution Therapy. These are all studied ways to get rid of faulty thoughts or force out traumatic events that get stuck in your brain.

About the Author

A.J. Otjen lives in Laurel, Montana. Originally from Oklahoma, Dr. Agnes J. Otjen has been a professor of marketing for over twenty years at Montana State University in Billings. Before becoming a professor, she was a marketing executive for over twenty years, in Colorado, Nevada, and Missouri. In addition to numerous newspaper and journal articles, A.J. has written, collaborated on, and published children's books that have been accepted by Indian Education for All in the Office of Public Instruction and chosen for award recognition in 2023 by the Library of Congress. This is A.J.'s first book of non-fiction.

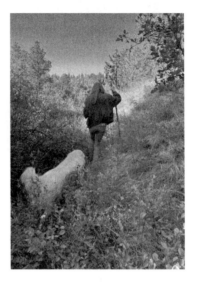